Osteoporosis Diet Cookbook for Seniors

Essential Recipes and Exercise Tips to Prevent Bone Loss, Strengthen Weak Bones, and Reduce Fracture Risk

OVIA COOPER

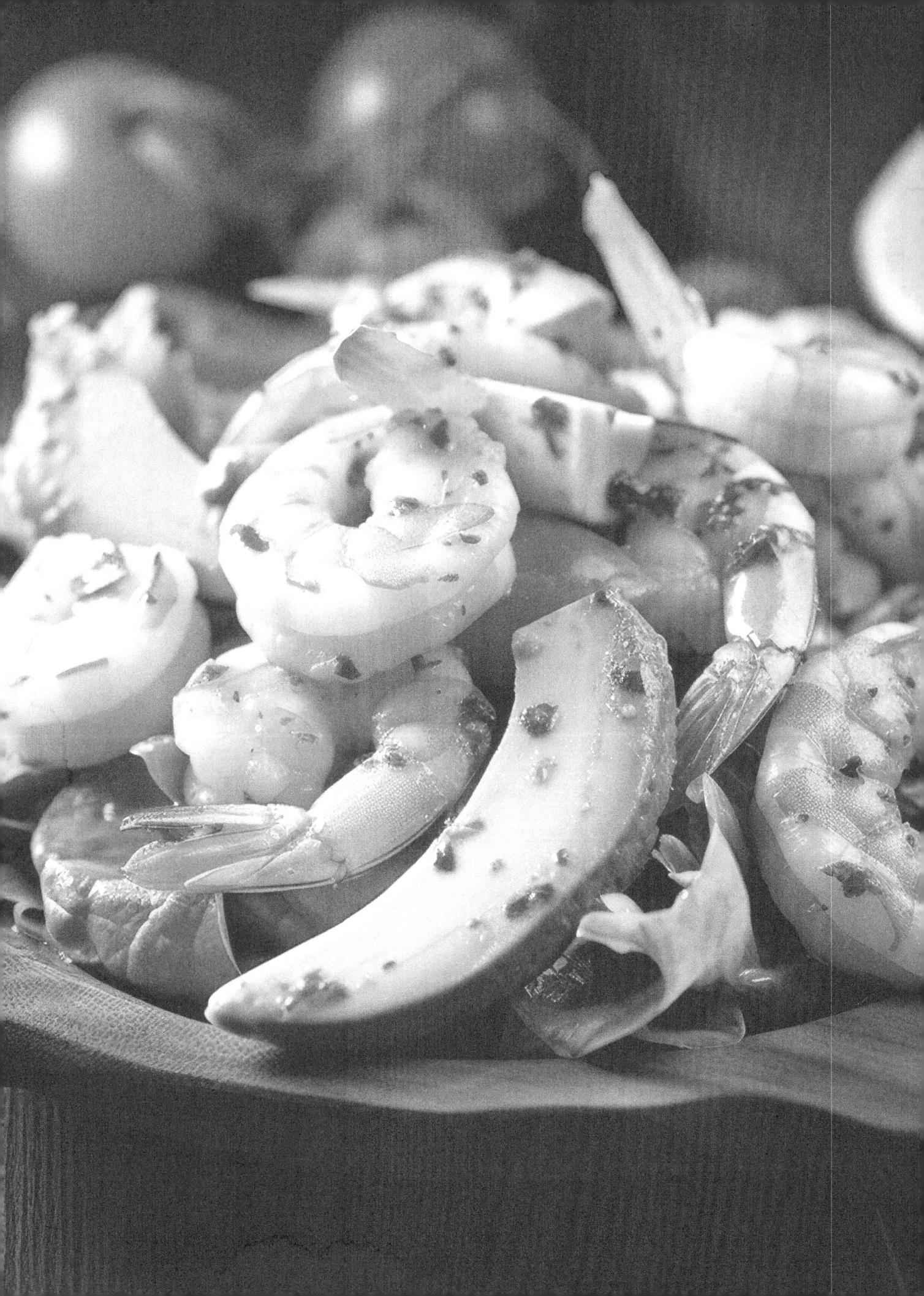

Copyright © 2024 by Ovia Cooper
All rights reserved.

No part of this publication may be reproduced, distributed, or transmitted in any form or by any means, including photocopying, recording, or other electronic or mechanical methods, without the prior written permission of the author, except in the case of brief quotations embodied in critical reviews and certain other noncommercial uses permitted by copyright law.

Disclaimer:

The content of this book is not intended to be a substitute for professional medical advice, diagnosis, or treatment. Always seek the advice of your physician or other qualified health providers with any questions you may have regarding a medical condition. Never disregard professional medical advice or delay in seeking it because of something you have read in this book.

ABOUT THE AUTHOR

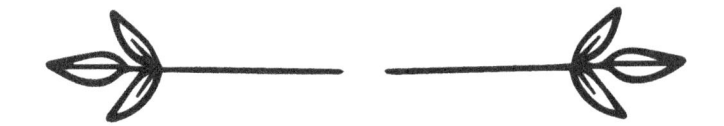

Ovia Cooper is a passionate advocate for senior health and wellness, drawing from personal experience to create impactful and transformative resources. With over two decades of dedication to nutrition and healthy living, Ovia understands the challenges that come with aging and the vital role diet plays in maintaining strength, vitality, and independence.

After facing her own struggles with osteoporosis, Ovia dedicated herself to learning everything she could about bone health. She discovered the power of nutrition as a tool for not just preventing bone loss but rebuilding and fortifying bones. Through her research and personal journey, Ovia has crafted a wealth of practical knowledge that she now shares with others.

In this book "Osteoporosis Diet Cookbook for Seniors," Ovia blends her expertise in nutrition with her love for simple, flavorful cooking. She believes that eating healthy doesn't need to be complicated or tasteless, and her recipes prove that you can enjoy every bite while nourishing your bones and body.

Ovia Cooper's writing is warm, relatable, and rooted in her own experiences, making her a trusted voice for seniors looking to regain control of their health. Her goal is simple: to help seniors live stronger, healthier, and more fulfilling lives through the power of good food.

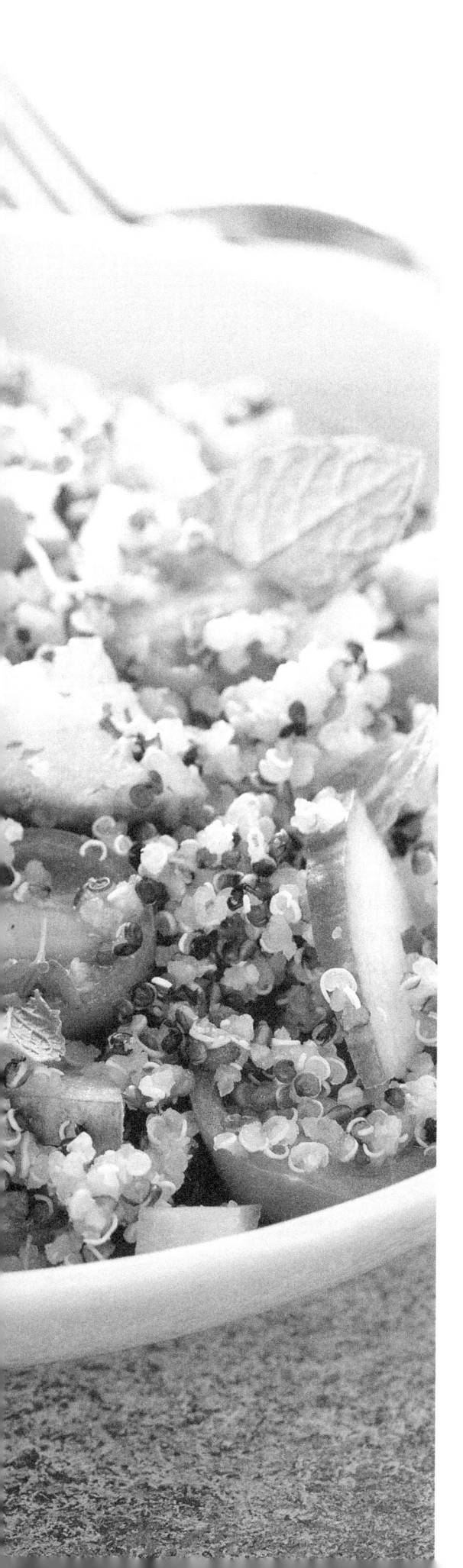

TABLE OF CONTENT

Introduction
- **Understanding Osteoporosis**
- **How Osteoporosis Affects Seniors**
- **Importance of Diet in Managing Osteoporosis**
- **Essential Nutrients for Bone Health**
- **Foods to Avoid for Better Bone Health**

7-9

Chapter 1: Calcium-Rich Breakfasts
- **Importance of Starting the Day with Calcium**
- **Quick and Easy Breakfast Recipes**

11-26

Chapter 2: Vitamin D-Packed Lunches
- **Recipes for Enhancing Bone Health Midday**

27-42

Chapter 3: Protein-Rich Dinners
- **Balancing Protein with Vegetables and Whole Grains**

43-56

Chapter 4: Bone-Boosting Snacks and Sides
- **Healthy Snacking Recipes for Bone Health**

57-64

Chapter 5: Delicious Calcium-Fortified Desserts
- **Calcium-Fortified Recipes as Guilt-Free Desserts**

65-72

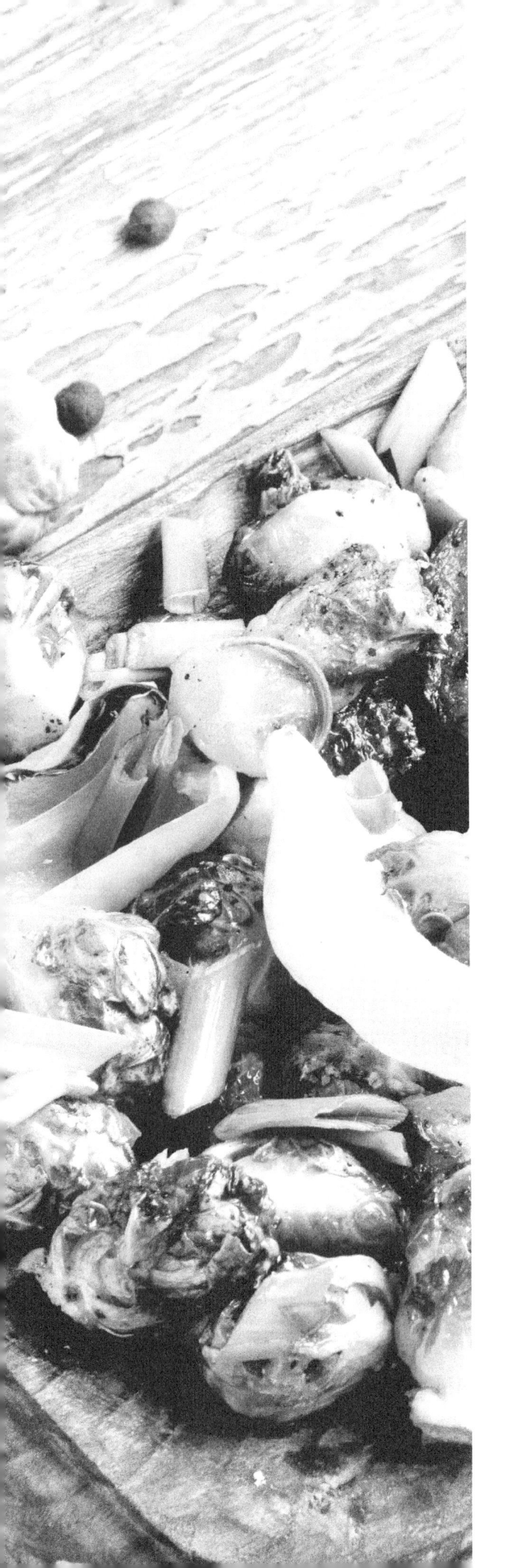

Chapter 6: Magnesium-Powered Meals **73-86**
- Role of Magnesium in Bone Density

Chapter 7: Meal Planning and Prep Tips for Seniors
- Simplifying Meal Preparation
- Budget-Friendly Shopping Tips for Bone-Healthy Foods
- Building Balanced Meals with Calcium and Vitamin D
- Portion Control for Seniors **87-90**
- Incorporating Seasonal Produce
- Meal Prep Tips for Busy Days
- Cooking on a Budget
- Smart Storage Solutions for Fresh Ingredients
- Easy-to-Cook Recipes for Caregivers

Chapter 8: Staying Active and Hydrated
- The Importance of Exercise in Supporting Bone Health **91-93**
- Hydration Tips for Seniors

Conclusion **95**

Bonus 1: 28 days Meal plan **97-100**

Bonus 2: Shopping List **101-104**

Appendix A: The Dity Dozen and the Clean Fifteen **105**

Appendix B: Conversion Tables **106-108**

INTRODUCTION

As a nutritionist and chef with over 20 years of experience, I've had the privilege of working with countless individuals, particularly seniors, to help them manage their health through diet. My journey began when I realized the profound impact that nutrition can have on conditions like osteoporosis—a condition that affects millions, particularly as they age.

Over the years, I've developed and fine-tuned recipes that not only nourish the body but also support bone health. I've seen firsthand how the right foods can strengthen bones, reduce the risk of fractures, and improve the overall quality of life for seniors. This cookbook is a culmination of my years of experience and passion for helping others live healthier, fuller lives. My goal is to provide you with the tools and knowledge you need to manage osteoporosis through delicious, nutrient-rich meals.

Understanding Osteoporosis
What is Osteoporosis?
Osteoporosis is a bone disease characterized by a decrease in bone mass and density, leading to fragile bones that are more prone to fractures. The term "osteoporosis" literally means "porous bones," and it's a condition that often goes unnoticed until a bone fracture occurs. The disease is particularly prevalent among seniors, especially women after menopause, due to the drop in estrogen levels, which is crucial for bone density maintenance.

How Osteoporosis Affects Seniors
As we get older, our bones gradually lose strength and density. However, for those with osteoporosis, this process is accelerated. The condition can lead to severe complications for seniors, including fractures from minor falls, particularly in the hip, spine, and wrist. Hip fractures are especially concerning as they can lead to long-term disability and even increase the risk of mortality. Osteoporosis can also cause a stooped posture and a reduction in height due to vertebral fractures.

Importance of Diet in Managing Osteoporosis

While genetics play a role in bone health, diet and lifestyle choices are crucial factors that can influence the progression of osteoporosis. A well-balanced diet rich in essential nutrients can help slow bone loss and may even improve bone density.

For seniors, maintaining bone health through diet is not just about preventing fractures but also about preserving independence, mobility, and overall well-being. This cookbook is designed to guide you in making dietary choices that will support your bone health without compromising on taste or enjoyment.

Essential Nutrients for Bone Health

- **Calcium**

Calcium is the building block of bones. About 99% of the body's calcium is stored in bones and teeth, providing structural support. For seniors, it's vital to consume enough calcium to prevent the body from leaching this mineral from the bones, leading to further bone loss.

Dairy products like milk, yogurt, and cheese are rich sources of calcium. However, for those who are lactose intolerant or prefer plant-based options, fortified plant milks, tofu, and leafy greens like kale and broccoli are excellent alternatives.

- **Vitamin D**

Vitamin D is essential for the absorption of calcium. Without adequate vitamin D, the body cannot absorb enough calcium, no matter how much is consumed. This vitamin is synthesized by the skin when exposed to sunlight, but as people age, the skin's ability to produce vitamin D decreases. Therefore, it's essential for seniors to include vitamin D-rich foods such as fatty fish (like salmon and mackerel), egg yolks, and fortified foods in their diet, or consider supplements if necessary.

- **Protein**

Protein is essential for tissue growth and repair, including the maintenance of healthy bones. It also helps maintain muscle mass, which is important for supporting and protecting bones. A diet with adequate protein from sources like poultry, fish, beans, legumes, and dairy can help ensure that bones remain strong and resilient.

- **Magnesium**

Magnesium plays a key role in bone formation and affects the function of osteoblasts and osteoclasts, the cells responsible for building and breaking down bone tissue. It also plays a role in converting vitamin D into its active form, which aids in calcium absorption. Foods like nuts, seeds, whole grains, and green leafy vegetables are rich in magnesium and should be included in a bone-healthy diet.

- **Vitamin K**

Vitamin K is vital for bone health as it helps in the regulation of calcium in the bones and aids in bone mineralization. It also plays a role in preventing the calcification of arteries and blood vessels, which is important for overall health. Leafy greens such as spinach, kale, and broccoli are rich sources of vitamin K.

Foods to Avoid for Better Bone Health

- **High-Sodium Foods**

A diet high in sodium can cause the body to lose calcium through urine, leading to bone loss. Seniors should be mindful of their sodium intake, particularly from processed and packaged foods, and aim to season meals with herbs and spices instead of salt.

- **Caffeine and Alcohol**

Excessive caffeine intake can interfere with calcium absorption, and alcohol can weaken bones and disrupt the balance of calcium in the body. It's important for seniors to limit their intake of caffeinated beverages like coffee and tea, and to drink alcohol in moderation, if at all.

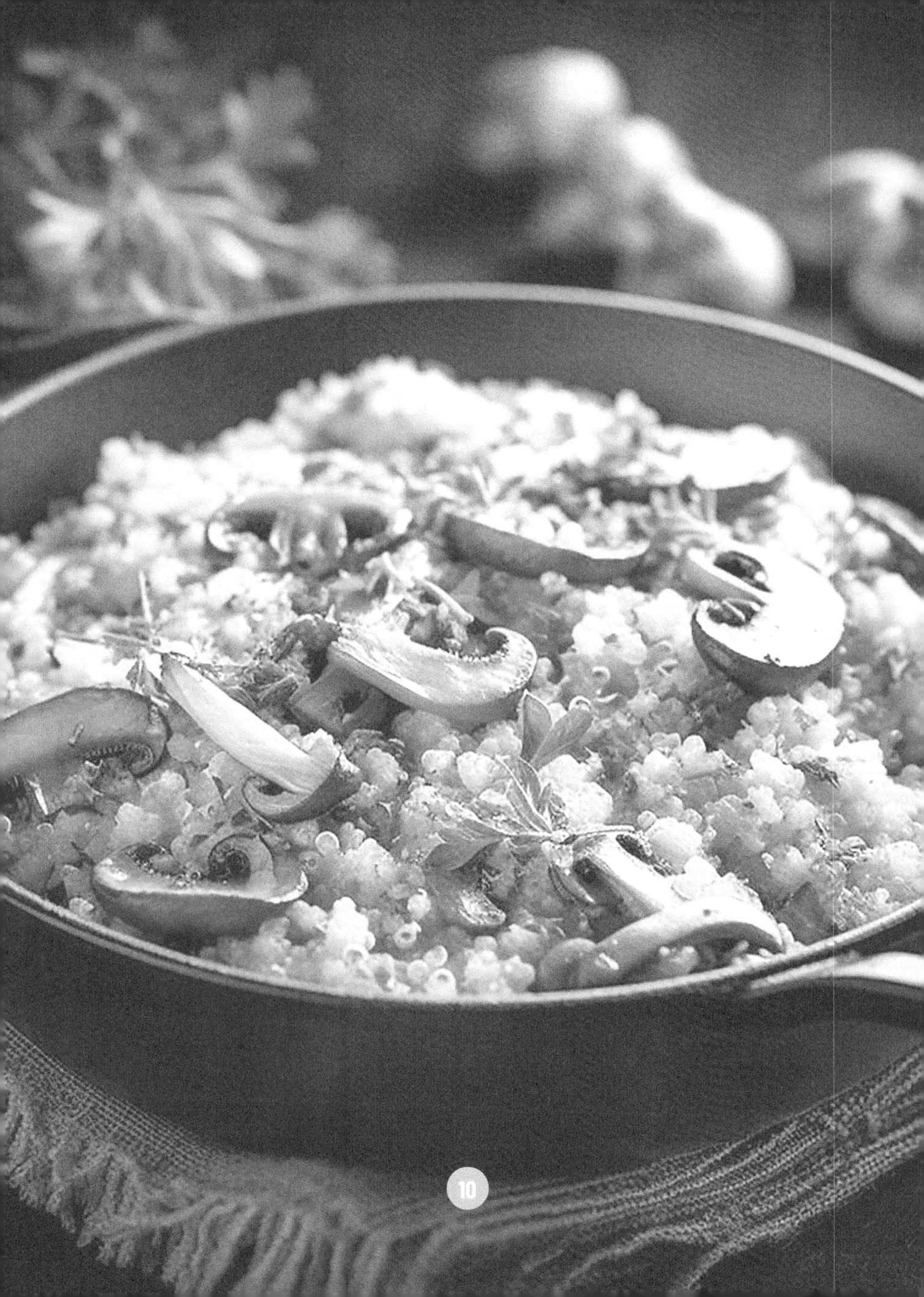

CHAPTER 1
Calcium-Rich Breakfasts

Starting your day with a calcium-rich breakfast is crucial for maintaining bone health, especially for seniors. Calcium plays a vital role in building and maintaining strong bones, and incorporating it into your morning routine ensures you're setting a strong foundation for the day ahead. The following recipes are designed to be quick, easy, and delicious, providing you with a nutritious start that supports your bone health.

Creamy Greek Yogurt Parfait with Berries and Nuts

Serves: 1, Prep Time: 5 minutes, Cook Time: 0 minutes, Total Time: 5 minutes
Calories: 250, Calcium: 300 mg, Protein: 15 g, Fat: 10 g, Carbohydrates: 28 g

Ingredients:
- 1 cup Greek yogurt (calcium-fortified if available)
- 1/2 cup mixed berries (strawberries, blueberries, raspberries)
- 2 tbsp chopped nuts (almonds, walnuts)
- 1 tbsp honey
- 1/4 cup granola

Instructions:
- In a glass or bowl, layer half of the Greek yogurt.
- Add a layer of mixed berries and then a sprinkle of chopped nuts.
- Drizzle with honey.
- Add the remaining Greek yogurt, another layer of berries, and top with granola.
- Enjoy immediately.

Spinach and Cheese Omelette

- **Serves:** 1
- **Prep Time:** 5 minutes
- **Cook Time:** 5 minutes
- **Total Time:** 10 minutes

Nutrition per serving:
- Calories: 220
- Calcium: 250 mg
- Protein: 18 g
- Fat: 15 g
- Carbohydrates: 4 g

Ingredients:
- 2 large eggs
- 1/4 cup shredded cheese (cheddar, mozzarella)
- 1/2 cup fresh spinach, chopped
- 1 tbsp milk (optional)
- Salt and pepper to taste
- 1 tsp olive oil

Instructions:
- In a bowl, beat the eggs with milk (if using), salt, and pepper.
- Heat olive oil in a non-stick pan over medium heat.
- Add the chopped spinach and cook until wilted.
- Pour the beaten eggs over the spinach.
- Sprinkle the shredded cheese over the eggs.
- Cook until the eggs are set, then fold the omelette in half.
- Serve hot.

Almond Milk and Chia Seed Pudding

- **Serves:** 1
- **Prep Time:** 5 minutes
- **Cook Time:** 0 minutes (requires 2 hours refrigeration)
- **Total Time:** 5 minutes + refrigeration time

Nutrition per serving:
- Calories: 200
- Calcium: 250 mg
- Protein: 6 g
- Fat: 11 g
- Carbohydrates: 19 g

Ingredients:
- 1 cup almond milk (calcium-fortified)
- 3 tbsp chia seeds
- 1 tbsp honey or maple syrup
- 1/2 tsp vanilla extract
- Fresh fruit for topping (optional)

Instructions:
- In a jar or bowl, mix almond milk, chia seeds, honey, and vanilla extract.
- Stir well and let sit for 5 minutes. Stir again to prevent clumping.
- Cover and refrigerate for at least 2 hours or overnight.
- Top with fresh fruit before serving.

Whole Grain Cereal with Fortified Milk

- **Serves:** 1
- **Prep Time:** 2 minutes
- **Cook Time:** 0 minutes
- **Total Time:** 2 minutes

Nutrition per serving:
- Calories: 300
- Calcium: 400 mg
- Protein: 12 g
- Fat: 5 g
- Carbohydrates: 55 g

Ingredients:
- 1 cup whole grain cereal
- 1 cup calcium-fortified milk (dairy or plant-based)
- 1/2 cup fresh fruit (optional)

Instructions:
- Pour the cereal into a bowl.
- Add the milk and stir.
- Top with fresh fruit if desired.
- Serve immediately.

Baked Oatmeal with Apples and Walnuts

- **Serves:** 4
- **Prep Time:** 10 minutes
- **Cook Time:** 35-40 minutes
- **Total Time:** 45-50 minutes

Ingredients:
- 1 cup rolled oats
- 1/2 cup apples, diced
- 1/4 cup walnuts, chopped
- 1 1/2 cups milk (calcium-fortified)
- 1/4 cup maple syrup or honey
- 1 tsp cinnamon
- 1/2 tsp baking powder
- 1/4 tsp salt
- 1 egg, beaten
- 1 tsp vanilla extract

Nutrition per serving:
- Calories: 350
- Calcium: 150 mg
- Protein: 8 g
- Fat: 15 g
- Carbohydrates: 45 g

Instructions:
- Preheat oven to 350°F (175°C).
- In a large bowl, combine oats, baking powder, cinnamon, and salt.
- In another bowl, mix the milk, egg, vanilla extract, and maple syrup.
- Pour the wet ingredients into the dry ingredients and stir until combined.
- Fold in the diced apples and walnuts.
- Pour the mixture into a greased baking dish.
- Bake for 35-40 minutes until the top is golden and the oatmeal is set.
- Let it cool slightly before serving.

Ricotta and Honey on Whole Grain Toast

- **Serves:** 1
- **Prep Time:** 3 minutes
- **Cook Time:** 2 minutes
- **Total Time:** 5 minutes

Nutrition per serving:
- Calories: 220
- Calcium: 200 mg
- Protein: 10 g
- Fat: 8 g
- Carbohydrates: 28 g

Ingredients:
- 1 slice whole grain bread, toasted
- 1/4 cup ricotta cheese
- 1 tsp honey
- 1/4 tsp ground cinnamon (optional)

Instructions:
1. Spread the ricotta cheese evenly over the toasted bread.
2. Drizzle with honey.
3. Sprinkle with ground cinnamon if desired.
4. Serve immediately.

Smoothie with Kale, Almond Butter, and Fortified Orange Juice

- **Serves:** 1
- **Prep Time:** 5 minutes
- **Cook Time:** 0 minutes
- **Total Time:** 5 minutes

Nutrition per serving:
- Calories: 250
- Calcium: 350 mg
- Protein: 8 g
- Fat: 12 g
- Carbohydrates: 30 g

Ingredients:
- 1 cup kale, chopped
- 1/2 banana
- 1 tbsp almond butter
- 1/2 cup calcium-fortified orange juice
- 1/2 cup almond milk (calcium-fortified)
- 1 tsp honey (optional)

Instructions:
- Combine all ingredients in a blender.
- Blend until smooth.
- Pour into a glass and enjoy immediately.

Scrambled Eggs with Spinach and Feta

- **Serves:** 1
- **Prep Time:** 5 minutes
- **Cook Time:** 5 minutes
- **Total Time:** 10 minutes

Nutrition per serving:
- Calories: 280
- Calcium: 220 mg
- Protein: 18 g
- Fat: 22 g
- Carbohydrates: 3 g

Ingredients:
- 2 large eggs
- 1/4 cup feta cheese, crumbled
- 1/2 cup fresh spinach, chopped
- 1 tbsp milk (optional)
- Salt and pepper to taste
- 1 tsp olive oil

Instructions:
- In a bowl, beat the eggs with milk (if using), salt, and pepper.
- Heat olive oil in a non-stick pan over medium heat.
- Add the chopped spinach and cook until wilted.
- Pour the beaten eggs over the spinach.
- Sprinkle the crumbled feta cheese over the eggs.
- Cook until the eggs are fully set, stirring occasionally.
- Serve hot.

Overnight Oats with Chia Seeds and Almonds

- **Serves:** 1
- **Prep Time:** 5 minutes
- **Cook Time:** 0 minutes (requires overnight refrigeration)
- **Total Time:** 5 minutes + refrigeration time

Nutrition per serving:
- Calories: 300
- Calcium: 250 mg
- Protein: 10 g
- Fat: 12 g
- Carbohydrates: 40 g

Ingredients:
- 1/2 cup rolled oats
- 1 tbsp chia seeds
- 1 tbsp chopped almonds
- 1 cup almond milk (calcium-fortified)
- 1 tbsp honey or maple syrup
- 1/2 tsp vanilla extract
- Fresh fruit for topping (optional)

Instructions:
- In a jar or bowl, combine oats, chia seeds, almonds, almond milk, honey, and vanilla extract.
- Stir well, cover, and refrigerate overnight.
- In the morning, stir the oats and top with fresh fruit if desired.
- Serve cold.

Quinoa Breakfast Bowl with Blueberries and Almonds

- **Serves:** 1
- **Prep Time:** 5 minutes
- **Cook Time:** 15 minutes (for cooking quinoa)
- **Total Time:** 20 minutes

Nutrition per serving:
- Calories: 320
- Calcium: 180 mg
- Protein: 12 g
- Fat: 10 g
- Carbohydrates: 50 g

Ingredients:
- 1/2 cup cooked quinoa
- 1/2 cup blueberries
- 1 tbsp chopped almonds
- 1/2 cup almond milk (calcium-fortified)
- 1 tbsp honey or maple syrup
- 1/4 tsp cinnamon (optional)

Instructions:
- In a bowl, combine cooked quinoa, blueberries, and almonds.
- Pour almond milk over the mixture.
- Drizzle with honey or maple syrup.
- Sprinkle with cinnamon if desired.
- Serve immediately.

Calcium-Fortified Pancakes with Maple Syrup

- **Serves:** 2
- **Prep Time:** 5 minutes
- **Cook Time:** 10 minutes
- **Total Time:** 15 minutes

Nutrition per serving:
- Calories: 300
- Calcium: 250 mg
- Protein: 8 g
- Fat: 10 g
- Carbohydrates: 40 g

Ingredients:
- 1 cup pancake mix (whole grain, if possible)
- 3/4 cup calcium-fortified milk (dairy or plant-based)
- 1 egg
- 1 tbsp vegetable oil or melted butter
- 1 tsp vanilla extract
- Maple syrup for serving

Instructions:
- In a bowl, mix the pancake mix, milk, egg, oil, and vanilla extract until smooth.
- Heat a non-stick skillet over medium heat and lightly grease it.
- Pour 1/4 cup of batter onto the skillet and cook until bubbles form on the surface.
- Flip the pancake and cook until golden brown on both sides.
- Serve with maple syrup.

Cottage Cheese with Pineapple and Walnuts

- **Serves:** 1
- **Prep Time:** 3 minutes
- **Cook Time:** 0 minutes
- **Total Time:** 3 minutes

Nutrition per serving:
- Calories: 300
- Calcium: 250 mg
- Protein: 8 g
- Fat: 10 g
- Carbohydrates: 40 g

Ingredients:
- 1/2 cup cottage cheese (low-fat, if preferred)
- 1/4 cup pineapple chunks (fresh or canned in juice)
- 1 tbsp chopped walnuts
- 1 tsp honey (optional)

Instructions:
- In a bowl, combine cottage cheese and pineapple chunks.
- Top with chopped walnuts.
- Drizzle with honey if desired.
- Serve immediately.

Tofu Scramble with Vegetables

- **Serves:** 1
- **Prep Time:** 5 minutes
- **Cook Time:** 10 minutes
- **Total Time:** 15 minutes

Nutrition per serving:
- Calories: 200
- Calcium: 300 mg
- Protein: 15 g
- Fat: 12 g
- Carbohydrates: 10 g

Ingredients:
- 1/2 block firm tofu, drained and crumbled
- 1/2 cup mixed vegetables (bell peppers, onions, spinach)
- 1 tbsp olive oil
- 1/2 tsp turmeric (for color)
- Salt and pepper to taste
- 1 tbsp nutritional yeast (optional)

Instructions:
- Heat olive oil in a skillet over medium heat.
- Add the mixed vegetables and cook until softened.
- Add the crumbled tofu, turmeric, salt, pepper, and nutritional yeast.
- Cook, stirring occasionally, until the tofu is heated through and resembles scrambled eggs.
- Serve hot.

Calcium-Fortified Waffles with Berry Compote

- **Serves:** 2
- **Prep Time:** 5 minutes
- **Cook Time:** 10 minutes
- **Total Time:** 15 minutes

Nutrition per serving:
- Calories: 320
- Calcium: 250 mg
- Protein: 10 g
- Fat: 12 g
- Carbohydrates: 42 g

Ingredients:
- 1 cup waffle mix (whole grain, if possible)
- 3/4 cup calcium-fortified milk (dairy or plant-based)
- 1 egg
- 1 tbsp vegetable oil or melted butter
- 1 tsp vanilla extract
- 1 cup mixed berries (fresh or frozen)
- 2 tbsp honey or maple syrup

Instructions:
- In a bowl, mix the waffle mix, milk, egg, oil, and vanilla extract until smooth.
- Preheat the waffle iron and lightly grease it.
- Pour the batter into the waffle iron and cook according to the manufacturer's instructions.
- Meanwhile, in a small saucepan, heat the berries with honey or maple syrup until warm and slightly thickened.
- Serve the waffles topped with berry compote.

Baked Egg Cups with Cheese and Spinach

- **Serves:** 4 (makes 8 egg cups)
- **Prep Time:** 5 minutes
- **Cook Time:** 15-20 minutes
- **Total Time:** 20-25 minutes

Nutrition per serving:
- Calories: 150
- Calcium: 180 mg
- Protein: 12 g
- Fat: 10 g
- Carbohydrates: 2 g

Ingredients:
- 4 large eggs
- 1/2 cup shredded cheese (cheddar, mozzarella)
- 1/2 cup fresh spinach, chopped
- Salt and pepper to taste
- 1 tsp olive oil

Instructions:
- Preheat the oven to 350°F (175°C).
- Lightly grease a muffin tin with olive oil.
- In a bowl, whisk the eggs with salt and pepper.
- Add the chopped spinach and shredded cheese to the egg mixture.
- Pour the mixture evenly into the muffin tin.
- Bake for 15-20 minutes, or until the egg cups are set.
- Let cool slightly before serving.

Fortified Almond Milk Latte with Whole Grain Muffin

- **Serves:** 1
- **Prep Time:** 5 minutes
- **Cook Time:** 5 minutes
- **Total Time:** 10 minutes

Nutrition per serving:
- Calories: 250
- Calcium: 200 mg
- Protein: 6 g
- Fat: 10 g
- Carbohydrates: 30 g

Ingredients:
- 1 cup almond milk (calcium-fortified)
- 1 shot of espresso or 1/2 cup strong brewed coffee
- 1 tsp honey or maple syrup
- 1 whole grain muffin (store-bought or homemade)

Instructions:
- Heat the almond milk until hot, but not boiling.
- Brew the espresso or coffee and pour it into a mug.
- Froth the almond milk (optional) and pour it over the coffee.
- Stir in honey or maple syrup if desired.
- Serve with a whole grain muffin.

CHAPTER 2
Vitamin D-Packed Lunches

Lunch is a crucial time to boost your vitamin D intake, essential for bone health and calcium absorption. The pairing of vitamin D-rich foods with calcium ensures your body effectively utilizes the calcium for strong bones.

Grilled Salmon Salad with Citrus Vinaigrette

Serves: 2, Prep Time: 10 minutes, Cook Time: 10 minutes, Total Time: 20 minutes
Calories: 350, Vitamin D: 500 IU, Protein: 25 g, Fat: 22 g, Carbohydrates: 10 g

Ingredients:
- 1 salmon fillet (4 oz)
- 4 cups mixed greens (spinach, arugula, romaine)
- 1/2 avocado, sliced
- 1/2 cup cherry tomatoes, halved
- 1/4 red onion, thinly sliced
- 1 orange, juiced (for vinaigrette)
- 2 tbsp olive oil (for vinaigrette)
- 1 tbsp lemon juice (for vinaigrette)
- Salt and pepper to taste

Instructions:
- Preheat the grill to medium-high heat.
- Season the salmon fillet with salt and pepper.
- Grill the salmon for 4-5 minutes on each side until cooked through.
- In a large bowl, combine the mixed greens, avocado, cherry tomatoes, and red onion.
- In a small bowl, whisk together the orange juice, olive oil, and lemon juice to make the vinaigrette.
- Top the salad with the grilled salmon and drizzle with the citrus vinaigrette.
- Serve immediately.

Mushroom and Tofu Stir-Fry

- **Serves:** 2
- **Prep Time:** 10 minutes
- **Cook Time:** 15 minutes
- **Total Time:** 25 minutes

Nutrition per serving:
- Calories: 250
- Vitamin D: 400 IU
- Protein: 15 g
- Fat: 12 g
- Carbohydrates: 20 g

Ingredients:
- 1 block firm tofu, cubed
- 2 cups mixed mushrooms (shiitake, button, cremini)
- 1 red bell pepper, sliced
- 2 tbsp soy sauce
- 1 tbsp sesame oil
- 1 tbsp olive oil
- 2 cloves garlic, minced
- 1 tsp ginger, minced
- 1 tbsp chopped green onions
- 1 tbsp sesame seeds (optional)

Instructions:
- Heat olive oil in a large skillet over medium heat.
- Add the cubed tofu and cook until golden brown on all sides. Remove and set aside.
- In the same skillet, add sesame oil, garlic, and ginger. Sauté until fragrant.
- Add the mushrooms and bell pepper, and stir-fry for 5-7 minutes until tender.
- Return the tofu to the skillet, and add soy sauce. Stir to combine.
- Cook for another 2 minutes, allowing the flavors to meld.
- Serve hot, garnished with green onions and sesame seeds.

Turkey and Avocado Wrap with Spinach

- **Serves:** 1
- **Prep Time:** 5 minutes
- **Cook Time:** 0 minutes
- **Total Time:** 5 minutes

Nutrition per serving:
- Calories: 350
- Vitamin D: 200 IU
- Protein: 20 g
- Fat: 18 g
- Carbohydrates: 30 g

Ingredients:
- 4 oz turkey breast, sliced
- 1 whole wheat tortilla
- 1/2 avocado, sliced
- 1 cup fresh spinach leaves
- 1 tbsp mayonnaise or Greek yogurt
- 1 tsp Dijon mustard
- Salt and pepper to taste

Instructions:
- Lay the tortilla flat and spread mayonnaise or Greek yogurt on it.
- Add Dijon mustard, then layer the turkey slices, avocado, and spinach.
- Season with salt and pepper.
- Roll up the tortilla tightly, securing it with toothpicks if necessary.
- Cut in half and serve immediately.

Egg Salad with Fresh Herbs

- **Serves:** 2
- **Prep Time:** 10 minutes
- **Cook Time:** 0 minutes (excluding time to boil eggs)
- **Total Time:** 10 minutes

Nutrition per serving:
- Calories: 300
- Vitamin D: 150 IU
- Protein: 15 g
- Fat: 22 g
- Carbohydrates: 5 g

Ingredients:
- 4 large eggs, hard-boiled and chopped
- 2 tbsp mayonnaise
- 1 tsp Dijon mustard
- 1 tbsp chopped fresh parsley
- 1 tbsp chopped fresh chives
- 1 tbsp chopped dill
- Salt and pepper to taste
- 2 slices whole grain bread (optional, for serving)

Instructions:
- In a medium bowl, combine the chopped eggs, mayonnaise, Dijon mustard, and fresh herbs.
- Mix well and season with salt and pepper.
- Serve on its own or spread over whole grain bread as a sandwich.

Sardine and Tomato Whole Grain Sandwich

- **Serves:** 1
- **Prep Time:** 5 minutes
- **Cook Time:** 0 minutes
- **Total Time:** 5 minutes

Nutrition per serving:
- Calories: 320
- Vitamin D: 350 IU
- Protein: 18 g
- Fat: 15 g
- Carbohydrates: 28 g

Ingredients:
- 1 can sardines in olive oil, drained
- 2 slices whole grain bread
- 1 tomato, sliced
- 1/4 red onion, thinly sliced
- 1 tbsp mayonnaise
- 1 tsp Dijon mustard
- Salt and pepper to taste
- Lettuce leaves (optional)

Instructions:
- In a small bowl, mash the sardines with mayonnaise and Dijon mustard.
- Spread the mixture evenly on one slice of bread.
- Top with tomato slices, red onion, and lettuce if using.
- Season with salt and pepper.
- Place the other slice of bread on top, cut in half, and serve.

Quinoa Salad with Kale and Grilled Chicken

- **Serves:** 2
- **Prep Time:** 10 minutes
- **Cook Time:** 15 minutes (for grilling chicken)
- **Total Time:** 25 minutes

Nutrition per serving:
- Calories: 400
- Vitamin D: 300 IU
- Protein: 30 g
- Fat: 15 g
- Carbohydrates: 35 g

Ingredients:
- 1/2 cup cooked quinoa
- 1 cup kale, chopped
- 1 grilled chicken breast, sliced
- 1/4 cup cherry tomatoes, halved
- 1/4 cup feta cheese, crumbled
- 2 tbsp olive oil
- 1 tbsp lemon juice
- Salt and pepper to taste

Instructions:
- In a large bowl, combine the cooked quinoa, kale, cherry tomatoes, and feta cheese.
- Add the sliced grilled chicken.
- In a small bowl, whisk together the olive oil and lemon juice.
- Pour the dressing over the salad and toss to combine.
- Season with salt and pepper, and serve.

Vitamin D-Fortified Soup with Chicken and Vegetables

- **Serves:** 4
- **Prep Time:** 10 minutes
- **Cook Time:** 25 minutes
- **Total Time:** 35 minutes

Nutrition per serving:

- Calories: 350
- Vitamin D: 400 IU
- Protein: 25 g
- Fat: 12 g
- Carbohydrates: 35 g

Ingredients:

- 1/2 lb chicken breast, cubed
- 2 cups mixed vegetables (carrots, celery, spinach)
- 4 cups chicken broth (vitamin D-fortified, if available)
- 1/2 cup barley or whole grain pasta
- 2 cloves garlic, minced
- 1 tbsp olive oil
- Salt and pepper to taste
- Fresh parsley for garnish

Instructions:

- Heat olive oil in a large pot over medium heat.
- Add the cubed chicken and cook until browned.
- Add the minced garlic and cook until fragrant.
- Add the chicken broth and bring to a boil.
- Stir in the vegetables and barley or pasta.
- Reduce the heat and simmer for 20-25 minutes until the grains are tender.
- Season with salt and pepper, and garnish with fresh parsley before serving.

Shrimp and Avocado Salad

- **Serves:** 2
- **Prep Time:** 10 minutes
- **Cook Time:** 0 minutes
- **Total Time:** 10 minutes

Nutrition per serving:
- Calories: 320
- Vitamin D: 300 IU
- Protein: 25 g
- Fat: 20 g
- Carbohydrates: 10 g

Ingredients:
- 8 oz cooked shrimp, peeled and deveined
- 1 avocado, diced
- 2 cups mixed greens (lettuce, spinach)
- 1/4 cup red onion, thinly sliced
- 1/2 cucumber, diced
- 2 tbsp olive oil
- 1 tbsp lemon juice
- 1 tsp Dijon mustard
- Salt and pepper to taste

Instructions:
- In a large bowl, combine the shrimp, avocado, mixed greens, red onion, and cucumber.
- In a small bowl, whisk together the olive oil, lemon juice, and Dijon mustard.
- Drizzle the dressing over the salad and toss to combine.
- Season with salt and pepper, and serve immediately.

Tuna Salad with Lemon and Dill

- **Serves:** 2
- **Prep Time:** 5 minutes
- **Cook Time:** 0 minutes
- **Total Time:** 5 minutes

Nutrition per serving:
- Calories: 250
- Vitamin D: 350 IU
- Protein: 30 g
- Fat: 10 g
- Carbohydrates: 5 g

Ingredients:
- 1 can tuna in water, drained
- 2 tbsp mayonnaise or Greek yogurt
- 1 tbsp lemon juice
- 1 tbsp fresh dill, chopped
- 1 celery stalk, diced
- 1/4 red onion, finely chopped
- Salt and pepper to taste
- Whole grain crackers or bread (optional, for serving)

Instructions:
- In a medium bowl, combine the tuna, mayonnaise or Greek yogurt, lemon juice, dill, celery, and red onion.
- Mix well and season with salt and pepper.
- Serve on its own or with whole grain crackers or bread.

Spinach and Mushroom Frittata

- **Serves:** 4
- **Prep Time:** 10 minutes
- **Cook Time:** 20 minutes
- **Total Time:** 30 minutes

Nutrition per serving:
- Calories: 280
- Vitamin D: 200 IU
- Protein: 20 g
- Fat: 18 g
- Carbohydrates: 10 g

Ingredients:
- 6 large eggs
- 1 cup fresh spinach, chopped
- 1 cup mushrooms, sliced
- 1/4 cup milk (optional)
- 1/4 cup shredded cheese (optional)
- 1 tbsp olive oil
- Salt and pepper to taste

Instructions:
- Preheat the oven to 350°F (175°C).
- In a large oven-safe skillet, heat the olive oil over medium heat.
- Add the mushrooms and sauté until soft, about 5 minutes.
- Add the spinach and cook until wilted.
- In a bowl, whisk the eggs with milk (if using), and season with salt and pepper.
- Pour the egg mixture into the skillet, spreading it evenly over the vegetables.
- Sprinkle cheese on top if desired.
- Transfer the skillet to the oven and bake for 15-20 minutes, or until the frittata is set.
- Let cool slightly before slicing and serving.

Roasted Veggie and Tofu Bowl

- **Serves:** 2
- **Prep Time:** 10 minutes
- **Cook Time:** 25 minutes
- **Total Time:** 35 minutes

Nutrition per serving:
- Calories: 350
- Vitamin D: 300 IU
- Protein: 20 g
- Fat: 18 g
- Carbohydrates: 30 g

Ingredients:
- 1 block firm tofu, cubed
- 2 cups mixed vegetables (broccoli, carrots, bell peppers)
- 1 tbsp olive oil
- 1 tbsp soy sauce
- 1 tsp garlic powder
- 1 tsp onion powder
- Salt and pepper to taste
- 1/2 cup cooked quinoa or brown rice

Instructions:
- Preheat the oven to 400°F (200°C).
- On a baking sheet, toss the tofu and vegetables with olive oil, soy sauce, garlic powder, onion powder, salt, and pepper.
- Roast in the oven for 20-25 minutes, until the vegetables are tender and the tofu is golden brown.
- Serve the roasted veggies and tofu over cooked quinoa or brown rice.

Smoked Salmon and Cucumber Sandwich

- **Serves:** 1
- **Prep Time:** 5 minutes
- **Cook Time:** 0 minutes
- **Total Time:** 5 minutes

Nutrition per serving:
- Calories: 300
- Vitamin D: 400 IU
- Protein: 18 g
- Fat: 15 g
- Carbohydrates: 25 g

Ingredients:
- 2 slices whole grain bread
- 3 oz smoked salmon
- 1/2 cucumber, thinly sliced
- 2 tbsp cream cheese
- 1 tsp capers (optional)
- Fresh dill for garnish

Instructions:
- Spread the cream cheese evenly on both slices of bread.
- Layer the smoked salmon and cucumber slices on one slice of bread.
- Sprinkle capers and fresh dill on top.
- Place the other slice of bread on top, cut in half, and serve.

Grilled Portobello Mushrooms with Quinoa

- **Serves:** 2
- **Prep Time:** 10 minutes
- **Cook Time:** 15 minutes
- **Total Time:** 25 minutes

Nutrition per serving:
- Calories: 320
- Vitamin D: 200 IU
- Protein: 15 g
- Fat: 10 g
- Carbohydrates: 45 g

Ingredients:
- 4 large portobello mushrooms, stems removed
- 1 cup cooked quinoa
- 2 tbsp olive oil
- 1 clove garlic, minced
- 1 tbsp balsamic vinegar
- Salt and pepper to taste
- Fresh parsley for garnish

Instructions:
- Preheat the grill to medium-high heat.
- Brush the mushrooms with olive oil and season with salt and pepper.
- Grill the mushrooms for 5-7 minutes on each side, until tender.
- In a small bowl, mix the minced garlic and balsamic vinegar with the cooked quinoa.
- Serve the grilled mushrooms topped with the quinoa mixture.
- Garnish with fresh parsley.

Chickpea and Spinach Salad with Sunflower Seeds

- **Serves:** 2
- **Prep Time:** 5 minutes
- **Cook Time:** 0 minutes
- **Total Time:** 5 minutes

Nutrition per serving:
- Calories: 300
- Vitamin D: 100 IU
- Protein: 12 g
- Fat: 18 g
- Carbohydrates: 28 g

Ingredients:
- 1 can chickpeas, drained and rinsed
- 2 cups fresh spinach, chopped
- 1/4 cup sunflower seeds
- 1/4 red onion, thinly sliced
- 2 tbsp olive oil
- 1 tbsp apple cider vinegar
- 1 tsp Dijon mustard
- Salt and pepper to taste

Instructions:
- In a large bowl, combine the chickpeas, spinach, sunflower seeds, and red onion.
- In a small bowl, whisk together the olive oil, apple cider vinegar, and Dijon mustard.
- Pour the dressing over the salad and toss to combine.
- Season with salt and pepper, and serve immediately.

Grilled Tilapia with Steamed Broccoli

- **Serves:** 2
- **Prep Time:** 5 minutes
- **Cook Time:** 10 minutes
- **Total Time:** 15 minutes

Nutrition per serving:

- Calories: 250
- Vitamin D: 250 IU
- Protein: 30 g
- Fat: 8 g
- Carbohydrates: 10 g

Ingredients:

- 2 tilapia fillets
- 1 tbsp olive oil
- 1 clove garlic, minced
- 1 lemon, juiced
- Salt and pepper to taste
- 2 cups broccoli florets

Instructions:

- Preheat the grill to medium-high heat.
- Brush the tilapia fillets with olive oil and season with minced garlic, lemon juice, salt, and pepper.
- Grill the fillets for 3-4 minutes on each side, until cooked through.
- Meanwhile, steam the broccoli until tender, about 5-7 minutes.
- Serve the grilled tilapia with the steamed broccoli on the side.

Baked Sweet Potato with Cottage Cheese and Chives

- **Serves:** 2
- **Prep Time:** 5 minutes
- **Cook Time:** 45 minutes
- **Total Time:** 50 minutes

Nutrition per serving:
- Calories: 280
- Vitamin D: 50 IU
- Protein: 10 g
- Fat: 5 g
- Carbohydrates: 50 g

Ingredients:
- 2 medium sweet potatoes
- 1/2 cup cottage cheese
- 2 tbsp fresh chives, chopped
- Salt and pepper to taste

Instructions:
- Preheat the oven to 400°F (200°C).
- Pierce the sweet potatoes with a fork and bake them directly on the oven rack for 45-50 minutes, or until tender.
- Cut the baked sweet potatoes in half and top with cottage cheese.
- Sprinkle with fresh chives, salt, and pepper before serving.

CHAPTER 3
Protein-Rich Dinners

- Protein is essential for maintaining muscle mass, which is particularly important for seniors as muscle loss can contribute to weakness and falls. Additionally, protein supports bone health by providing the necessary building blocks for bone tissue.
- Incorporating a variety of vegetables and whole grains with protein-rich foods ensures a balanced meal that supports overall health and well-being.

Roasted Chicken with Quinoa and Steamed Broccoli

Serves: 2, Prep Time: 10 minutes, Cook Time: 30 minutes, Total Time: 40 minutes
Calories: 450, Protein: 35 g, Fat: 15 g, Carbohydrates: 40 g

Ingredients:
- 2 chicken breasts
- 1 cup quinoa
- 2 cups broccoli florets
- 2 tbsp olive oil
- 1 clove garlic, minced
- 1 lemon, juiced
- Salt and pepper to taste

Instructions:
- Preheat the oven to 375°F (190°C).
- Rub the chicken breasts with olive oil, minced garlic, lemon juice, salt, and pepper.
- Place the chicken on a baking sheet and roast for 25-30 minutes, or until cooked through.
- Meanwhile, cook the quinoa according to the package instructions.
- Steam the broccoli until tender, about 5-7 minutes.
- Serve the roasted chicken with quinoa and steamed broccoli on the side.

Lentil and Vegetable Stew

- **Serves:** 4
- **Prep Time:** 10 minutes
- **Cook Time:** 35 minutes
- **Total Time:** 45 minutes

Nutrition per serving:
- Calories: 350
- Protein: 18 g
- Fat: 8 g
- Carbohydrates: 55 g

Ingredients:
- 1 cup dried lentils, rinsed
- 1 onion, diced
- 2 carrots, diced
- 2 celery stalks, diced
- 2 cups diced tomatoes
- 4 cups vegetable broth
- 2 tbsp olive oil
- 1 tsp cumin
- 1 tsp paprika
- Salt and pepper to taste

Instructions:
- In a large pot, heat olive oil over medium heat.
- Add the onion, carrots, and celery, and sauté until softened, about 5 minutes.
- Stir in the lentils, diced tomatoes, and vegetable broth.
- Add cumin, paprika, salt, and pepper.
- Bring to a boil, then reduce heat and simmer for 30-35 minutes, until lentils are tender.
- Serve hot, garnished with fresh herbs if desired.

Grilled Tofu with Stir-Fried Vegetables

- **Serves:** 2
- **Prep Time:** 10 minutes
- **Cook Time:** 15 minutes
- **Total Time:** 25 minutes

Nutrition per serving:
- Calories: 320
- Protein: 20 g
- Fat: 15 g
- Carbohydrates: 30 g

Ingredients:
- 1 block firm tofu, pressed and sliced
- 2 cups mixed vegetables (bell peppers, zucchini, mushrooms)
- 2 tbsp soy sauce
- 1 tbsp sesame oil
- 1 tsp ginger, minced
- 1 tsp garlic, minced
- 1 tbsp sesame seeds for garnish

Instructions:
- Preheat the grill to medium heat.
- Brush the tofu slices with sesame oil and grill for 3-4 minutes on each side, until golden.
- In a large pan, heat the remaining sesame oil and sauté the garlic and ginger until fragrant.
- Add the mixed vegetables and stir-fry for 5-7 minutes, until tender-crisp.
- Stir in the soy sauce and cook for another 2 minutes.
- Serve the grilled tofu on a plate with stir-fried vegetables and garnish with sesame seeds.

Baked Cod with Sweet Potato and Asparagus

- **Serves:** 2
- **Prep Time:** 10 minutes
- **Cook Time:** 30 minutes
- **Total Time:** 40 minutes

Nutrition per serving:
- Calories: 380
- Protein: 30 g
- Fat: 12 g
- Carbohydrates: 40 g

Ingredients:
- 2 cod fillets
- 2 medium sweet potatoes, peeled and cubed
- 1 bunch asparagus, trimmed
- 2 tbsp olive oil
- 1 lemon, juiced
- 1 tsp thyme
- Salt and pepper to taste

Instructions:
- Preheat the oven to 400°F (200°C).
- Toss the sweet potatoes with 1 tbsp olive oil, thyme, salt, and pepper, and spread them on a baking sheet.
- Bake for 15 minutes, then add the asparagus to the baking sheet.
- Drizzle the cod fillets with the remaining olive oil and lemon juice, and season with salt and pepper.
- Place the cod on the baking sheet with the vegetables and bake for an additional 12-15 minutes, until the fish is opaque and flakes easily with a fork.
- Serve the cod with sweet potato and asparagus.

Beef and Vegetable Stir-Fry with Brown Rice

- **Serves:** 2
- **Prep Time:** 10 minutes
- **Cook Time:** 15 minutes
- **Total Time:** 25 minutes

Nutrition per serving:

- Calories: 450
- Protein: 30 g
- Fat: 15 g
- Carbohydrates: 50 g

Ingredients:

- 8 oz beef sirloin, thinly sliced
- 2 cups mixed vegetables (broccoli, bell peppers, carrots)
- 2 cups cooked brown rice
- 2 tbsp soy sauce
- 1 tbsp oyster sauce
- 1 tbsp vegetable oil
- 1 clove garlic, minced
- 1 tsp ginger, minced

Instructions:

- In a large pan, heat the vegetable oil over medium-high heat.
- Add the garlic and ginger, and stir-fry until fragrant.
- Add the beef slices and cook for 2-3 minutes, until browned.
- Add the mixed vegetables and stir-fry for another 5-7 minutes, until the vegetables are tender.
- Stir in the soy sauce and oyster sauce, and cook for an additional 2 minutes.
- Serve the stir-fry over brown rice.

Stuffed Bell Peppers with Quinoa and Ground Turkey

- **Serves:** 4
- **Prep Time:** 15 minutes
- **Cook Time:** 30 minutes
- **Total Time:** 45 minutes

Nutrition per serving:
- Calories: 380
- Protein: 28 g
- Fat: 10 g
- Carbohydrates: 45 g

Ingredients:
- 4 large bell peppers, tops cut off and seeds removed
- 1 cup cooked quinoa
- 1/2 lb ground turkey
- 1 onion, diced
- 1 clove garlic, minced
- 1 can diced tomatoes
- 1 tsp cumin
- 1 tsp paprika
- Salt and pepper to taste
- 1/4 cup shredded cheese (optional)

Instructions:
- Preheat the oven to 375°F (190°C).
- In a large pan, cook the ground turkey over medium heat until browned.
- Add the onion and garlic, and sauté until softened.
- Stir in the cooked quinoa, diced tomatoes, cumin, paprika, salt, and pepper.
- Stuff the bell peppers with the quinoa and turkey mixture, and place them in a baking dish.
- Sprinkle the tops with shredded cheese if desired.
- Bake for 25-30 minutes, until the peppers are tender.

Grilled Shrimp Skewers with Veggie Couscous

- **Serves:** 2
- **Prep Time:** 10 minutes
- **Cook Time:** 10 minutes
- **Total Time:** 20 minutes

Nutrition per serving:
- Calories: 400
- Protein: 28 g
- Fat: 12 g
- Carbohydrates: 50 g

Ingredients:
- 12 large shrimp, peeled and deveined
- 1 cup couscous
- 1 cup mixed vegetables (zucchini, bell peppers, cherry tomatoes)
- 2 tbsp olive oil
- 1 tsp garlic powder
- 1 tsp paprika
- 1 lemon, juiced
- Salt and pepper to taste

Instructions:
- Preheat the grill to medium heat.
- Thread the shrimp onto skewers and brush with olive oil, garlic powder, paprika, lemon juice, salt, and pepper.
- Grill the shrimp skewers for 2-3 minutes on each side, until pink and cooked through.
- Cook the couscous according to the package instructions.
- In a large pan, sauté the mixed vegetables in olive oil until tender, about 5 minutes.
- Stir the vegetables into the cooked couscous and serve alongside the grilled shrimp skewers.

Vegetarian Chili with Black Beans and Sweet Corn

- **Serves:** 4
- **Prep Time:** 10 minutes
- **Cook Time:** 25 minutes
- **Total Time:** 35 minutes

Nutrition per serving:
- Calories: 340
- Protein: 15 g
- Fat: 8 g
- Carbohydrates: 60 g

Ingredients:
- 1 can black beans, drained and rinsed
- 1 can diced tomatoes
- 1 cup sweet corn (frozen or fresh)
- 1 onion, diced
- 2 cloves garlic, minced
- 1 tbsp chili powder
- 1 tsp cumin
- 1 tsp paprika
- 2 cups vegetable broth
- 1 tbsp olive oil
- Salt and pepper to taste

Instructions:
- In a large pot, heat olive oil over medium heat.
- Add the onion and garlic, and sauté until softened, about 5 minutes.
- Stir in the chili powder, cumin, and paprika, and cook for 1 minute to release the flavors.
- Add the black beans, diced tomatoes, sweet corn, and vegetable broth.
- Bring to a boil, then reduce heat and simmer for 20-25 minutes, until the chili thickens.
- Season with salt and pepper to taste and serve hot.

Herb-Crusted Pork Tenderloin with Roasted Root Vegetables

- **Serves:** 4
- **Prep Time:** 15 minutes
- **Cook Time:** 30 minutes
- **Total Time:** 45 minutes

Nutrition per serving:
- Calories: 450
- Protein: 35 g
- Fat: 18 g
- Carbohydrates: 40 g

Ingredients:
- 1 lb pork tenderloin
- 1 tbsp fresh rosemary, chopped
- 1 tbsp fresh thyme, chopped
- 2 tbsp olive oil
- 2 cloves garlic, minced
- 2 carrots, peeled and chopped
- 2 parsnips, peeled and chopped
- 2 sweet potatoes, peeled and cubed
- Salt and pepper to taste

Instructions:
- Preheat the oven to 400°F (200°C).
- In a small bowl, mix rosemary, thyme, minced garlic, salt, and pepper with 1 tbsp olive oil.
- Rub the herb mixture over the pork tenderloin.
- In a separate bowl, toss the root vegetables with the remaining olive oil, salt, and pepper.
- Place the pork tenderloin on a baking sheet and arrange the root vegetables around it.
- Roast for 25-30 minutes, until the pork reaches an internal temperature of 145°F (63°C).
- Let the pork rest for 5 minutes before slicing and serving with the roasted vegetables.

Spaghetti with Turkey Meatballs and Marinara Sauce

- **Serves:** 4
- **Prep Time:** 15 minutes
- **Cook Time:** 25 minutes
- **Total Time:** 40 minutes

Nutrition per serving:
- Calories: 500
- Protein: 30 g
- Fat: 15 g
- Carbohydrates: 60 g

Ingredients:
- 1 lb ground turkey
- 1/4 cup breadcrumbs
- 1/4 cup grated Parmesan cheese
- 1 egg, beaten
- 2 cloves garlic, minced
- 1 tsp Italian seasoning
- Salt and pepper to taste
- 2 cups marinara sauce
- 8 oz whole grain spaghetti
- 2 tbsp olive oil
- Fresh basil for garnish (optional)

Instructions:
- Preheat the oven to 375°F (190°C).
- In a large bowl, combine the ground turkey, breadcrumbs, Parmesan cheese, beaten egg, minced garlic, Italian seasoning, salt, and pepper.
- Form the mixture into meatballs and place them on a baking sheet.
- Bake the meatballs for 20-25 minutes, until cooked through.
- Meanwhile, cook the spaghetti according to package instructions.
- In a large pan, heat the marinara sauce over medium heat and add the cooked meatballs.
- Serve the meatballs and marinara sauce over the spaghetti, garnished with fresh basil if desired.

Baked Eggplant Parmesan with Whole Grain Pasta

- **Serves:** 4
- **Prep Time:** 15 minutes
- **Cook Time:** 25 minutes
- **Total Time:** 40 minutes

Nutrition per serving:
- Calories: 480
- Protein: 20 g
- Fat: 18 g
- Carbohydrates: 60 g

Ingredients:
- 1 large eggplant, sliced into rounds
- 1 cup marinara sauce
- 1 cup shredded mozzarella cheese
- 1/4 cup grated Parmesan cheese
- 1 cup whole grain breadcrumbs
- 1 egg, beaten
- 8 oz whole grain pasta
- 2 tbsp olive oil
- Fresh basil for garnish (optional)

Instructions:
- Preheat the oven to 375°F (190°C).
- Dip the eggplant slices into the beaten egg, then coat with breadcrumbs.
- In a large pan, heat the olive oil over medium heat and fry the eggplant slices until golden on both sides.
- In a baking dish, layer the fried eggplant slices, marinara sauce, and shredded mozzarella cheese.
- Sprinkle the top with grated Parmesan cheese and bake for 20-25 minutes, until bubbly and golden.
- Meanwhile, cook the whole grain pasta according to package instructions.
- Serve the baked eggplant Parmesan over the pasta, garnished with fresh basil if desired.

Chicken and Broccoli Stir-Fry with Brown Rice

- **Serves:** 4
- **Prep Time:** 10 minutes
- **Cook Time:** 15 minutes
- **Total Time:** 25 minutes

Nutrition per serving:
- Calories: 420
- Protein: 28 g
- Fat: 10 g
- Carbohydrates: 55 g

Ingredients:
- 1 lb chicken breast, sliced into strips
- 2 cups broccoli florets
- 1 cup brown rice
- 2 cloves garlic, minced
- 2 tbsp soy sauce
- 1 tbsp sesame oil
- 1 tbsp olive oil
- 1 tsp cornstarch mixed with 2 tbsp water (optional, for thickening sauce)
- Salt and pepper to taste

Instructions:
- Cook the brown rice according to package instructions.
- In a large pan, heat olive oil over medium-high heat and stir-fry the chicken strips until browned and cooked through, about 5-7 minutes.
- Remove the chicken from the pan and set aside.
- In the same pan, add sesame oil and garlic, and sauté for 1 minute.
- Add the broccoli florets and stir-fry for 3-4 minutes, until tender-crisp.
- Return the chicken to the pan and add soy sauce, stirring to coat.
- If a thicker sauce is desired, stir in the cornstarch mixture and cook for an additional 1-2 minutes until the sauce thickens.
- Serve the stir-fry over brown rice.

Quinoa-Stuffed Zucchini Boats

- **Serves:** 4
- **Prep Time:** 15 minutes
- **Cook Time:** 25 minutes
- **Total Time:** 40 minutes

Nutrition per serving:
- Calories: 380
- Protein: 14 g
- Fat: 15 g
- Carbohydrates: 50 g

Ingredients:
- 4 medium zucchini, halved lengthwise
- 1 cup cooked quinoa
- 1/2 cup diced tomatoes
- 1/2 cup black beans, drained and rinsed
- 1/2 cup corn kernels (fresh or frozen)
- 1/2 cup shredded cheddar cheese
- 1/4 cup chopped fresh cilantro
- 2 tbsp olive oil
- 1 tsp cumin
- Salt and pepper to taste

Instructions:
- Preheat the oven to 375°F (190°C).
- Scoop out the center of each zucchini half to create a boat shape, and place them on a baking sheet.
- In a large bowl, combine the cooked quinoa, diced tomatoes, black beans, corn kernels, cumin, salt, and pepper.
- Fill each zucchini boat with the quinoa mixture and top with shredded cheddar cheese.
- Drizzle the zucchini boats with olive oil.
- Bake for 20-25 minutes, until the zucchini is tender and the cheese is melted and bubbly.
- Garnish with chopped fresh cilantro before serving.

Miso Soup with Tofu and Seaweed

Serves: 4, Prep Time: 15 minutes, Cook Time: 25 minutes, Total Time: 40 minutes

Calories: 120, Protein: 8 g, Fat: 5 g, Carbohydrates: 12 g

Ingredients:
- 4 cups water
- 1/4 cup miso paste
- 1 cup tofu, cubed
- 1/4 cup dried seaweed
- 2 green onions, sliced
- 1 tbsp soy sauce
- 1 tsp sesame oil

Instructions:
- In a large pot, bring the water to a simmer.
- Whisk in the miso paste until fully dissolved.
- Add the cubed tofu and dried seaweed, and cook for 5 minutes.
- Stir in the soy sauce and sesame oil.
- Garnish with sliced green onions before serving.

Salmon with Wild Rice and Green Beans

Serves: 2, Prep Time: 10 minutes, Cook Time: 20 minutes, Total Time: 30 minutes

Calories: 450, Protein: 30 g, Fat: 18 g, Carbohydrates: 40 g

Ingredients:
- 2 salmon fillets
- 1 cup wild rice
- 2 cups green beans, trimmed
- 2 tbsp olive oil
- 1 lemon, juiced
- 1 clove garlic, minced
- Salt and pepper to taste

Instructions:
- Preheat the oven to 375°F (190°C).
- Rub the salmon fillets with olive oil, minced garlic, lemon juice, salt, and pepper.
- Place the salmon on a baking sheet and bake for 15-20 minutes, until the fish is opaque and flakes easily with a fork.
- Meanwhile, cook the wild rice according to package instructions.
- Steam the green beans until tender, about 5-7 minutes.
- Serve the salmon with wild rice and green beans on the side.

CHAPTER 4
Bone-Boosting Snacks and Sides

- Snacking can be a great opportunity to incorporate nutrient-rich foods that support bone health, especially when these snacks are packed with calcium, vitamin D, protein, and other essential nutrients.
- Complementing meals with nutrient-dense sides can ensure a balanced diet that promotes strong bones.

Kale Chips with Sea Salt

- Serves: 4
- Prep Time: 5 minutes
- Cook Time: 20 minutes
- Total Time: 25 minutes

Nutrition per serving:
- Calories: 50
- Protein: 2 g
- Fat: 2 g
- Carbohydrates: 8 g

Ingredients:
- 1 bunch kale, stems removed and leaves torn into bite-sized pieces
- 1 tbsp olive oil
- 1/2 tsp sea salt

Instructions:
- Preheat the oven to 300°F (150°C).
- Toss the kale leaves in olive oil and sea salt.
- Spread the kale on a baking sheet in a single layer.
- Bake for 15-20 minutes, turning halfway through, until crispy.
- Let cool and enjoy as a crunchy snack.

Cottage Cheese and Pineapple Bowl

Serves: 2, Prep Time: 5 minutes, Total Time: 5 minutes

Calories: 180, Protein: 14 g, Fat: 5 g, Carbohydrates: 24 g

Ingredients:
- 4 cups water
- 1/4 cup miso paste
- 1 cup tofu, cubed
- 1/4 cup dried seaweed
- 2 green onions, sliced
- 1 tbsp soy sauce
- 1 tsp sesame oil

Instructions:
- In a large pot, bring the water to a simmer.
- Whisk in the miso paste until fully dissolved.
- Add the cubed tofu and dried seaweed, and cook for 5 minutes.
- Stir in the soy sauce and sesame oil.
- Garnish with sliced green onions before serving.

Roasted Almonds and Dried Fruit Mix

Serves: 4, Prep Time: 5 minutes, Cook Time: 12 minutes, Total Time: 17 minutes

Calories: 220, Protein: 6 g, Fat: 14 g, Carbohydrates: 20 g

Ingredients:
- 1 cup raw almonds
- 1/2 cup dried cranberries
- 1/2 cup dried apricots, chopped

Instructions:
- Preheat the oven to 350°F (175°C).
- Spread the almonds on a baking sheet and roast for 10-12 minutes until golden.
- Allow the almonds to cool, then mix with dried cranberries and chopped apricots.
- Store in an airtight container for a quick and healthy snack.

Garlic and Parmesan Roasted Brussels Sprouts

Serves: 4, Prep Time: 10 minutes, Cook Time: 25 minutes, Total Time: 35 minutes

Calories: 140, Protein: 6 g, Fat: 9 g, Carbohydrates: 12 g

Ingredients:
- 1 lb Brussels sprouts, trimmed and halved
- 2 tbsp olive oil
- 2 cloves garlic, minced
- 1/4 cup grated Parmesan cheese
- Salt and pepper to taste

Instructions:
- Preheat the oven to 400°F (200°C).
- Toss the Brussels sprouts with olive oil, garlic, salt, and pepper.
- Spread the sprouts on a baking sheet in a single layer.
- Roast for 20-25 minutes until golden and crispy, turning halfway through.
- Remove from the oven and sprinkle with Parmesan cheese before serving.

Hummus with Carrot and Cucumber Sticks

Serves: 4, Prep Time: 5 minutes, Total Time: 5 minutes

Calories: 150, Protein: 4 g, Fat: 10 g, Carbohydrates: 12 g

Ingredients:
- 1 cup hummus (store-bought or homemade)
- 2 large carrots, cut into sticks
- 1 cucumber, cut into sticks

Instructions:
- Arrange the carrot and cucumber sticks on a plate.
- Serve with hummus for dipping.

Greek Yogurt with Honey and Granola

Serves: 1, Prep Time: 3 minutes, Total Time: 3 minutes

Calories: 200, Protein: 10 g, Fat: 5 g, Carbohydrates: 30 g

Ingredients:
- 1 cup Greek yogurt
- 1 tbsp honey
- 1/4 cup granola

Instructions:
- In a bowl, spoon the Greek yogurt.
- Drizzle with honey and top with granola.
- Serve immediately.

Sliced Apple with Almond Butter

Serves: 1, Prep Time: 3 minutes, Total Time: 3 minutes

Calories: 190, Protein: 4 g, Fat: 9 g, Carbohydrates: 26 g

Ingredients:
- 1 apple, sliced
- 2 tbsp almond butter

Instructions:
- Arrange the apple slices on a plate.
- Serve with almond butter for dipping.

Edamame with Sea Salt

Serves: 2, Prep Time: 5 minutes, Cook Time: 5 minutes, Total Time: 10 minutes

Calories: 120, Protein: 11 g, Fat: 5 g, Carbohydrates: 9 g

Ingredients:
- 1 cup shelled edamame (fresh or frozen)
- 1/2 tsp sea salt

Instructions:
- Cook the edamame according to package instructions.
- Sprinkle with sea salt and serve warm.

Cheese and Whole Grain Crackers

Serves: 1, Prep Time: 2 minutes, Total Time: 2 minutes

Calories: 180, Protein: 7 g, Fat: 10 g, Carbohydrates: 16 g

Ingredients:
- 2 oz cheese (cheddar, mozzarella, or your choice)
- 8 whole grain crackers

Instructions:
- Slice the cheese and arrange it with whole grain crackers on a plate.
- Serve immediately.

Baked Sweet Potato Fries

Serves: 4, Prep Time: 10 minutes, Cook Time: 30 minutes, Total Time: 40 minutes

Calories: 170, Protein: 2 g, Fat: 7 g, Carbohydrates: 26 g

Ingredients:
- 2 large sweet potatoes, peeled and cut into fries
- 2 tbsp olive oil
- 1/2 tsp paprika
- Salt and pepper to taste

Instructions:
- Preheat the oven to 425°F (220°C).
- Toss the sweet potato fries with olive oil, paprika, salt, and pepper.
- Spread the fries on a baking sheet in a single layer.
- Bake for 25-30 minutes, turning halfway through, until crispy and golden.
- Serve immediately.

Vegetable Crudité with Yogurt Dip

Serves: 4, Prep Time: 10 minutes, Total Time: 10 minutes

Calories: 100, Protein: 5 g, Fat: 4 g, Carbohydrates: 12 g

Ingredients:

- 1 cup plain Greek yogurt
- 1 tbsp lemon juice
- 1 tsp garlic powder
- 1 tsp dill, chopped
- Salt and pepper to taste
- Assorted vegetables (carrots, cucumbers, bell peppers, cherry tomatoes) cut into sticks

Instructions:

- In a small bowl, mix Greek yogurt with lemon juice, garlic powder, dill, salt, and pepper.
- Arrange the vegetable sticks on a platter and serve with the yogurt dip.

Spinach and Artichoke Dip with Whole Grain Pita

Serves: 4, Prep Time: 10 minutes, Cook Time: 25 minutes, Total Time: 35 minutes

Calories: 180, Protein: 6 g, Fat: 10 g, Carbohydrates: 18 g

Ingredients:

- 1 cup fresh spinach, chopped
- 1/2 cup canned artichoke hearts, chopped
- 1/4 cup low-fat cream cheese
- 1/4 cup Greek yogurt
- 1/4 cup grated Parmesan cheese
- 1 clove garlic, minced
- Salt and pepper to taste
- Whole grain pita, cut into wedges

Instructions:

- Preheat the oven to 375°F (190°C).
- In a bowl, mix spinach, artichoke hearts, cream cheese, Greek yogurt, Parmesan cheese, garlic, salt, and pepper.
- Transfer the mixture to a small baking dish.
- Bake for 20-25 minutes until the dip is hot and bubbly.
- Serve with whole grain pita wedges.

Roasted Chickpeas with Paprika

Serves: 4, Prep Time: 5 minutes, Cook Time: 30 minutes, Total Time: 35 minutes

Calories: 130, Protein: 6 g, Fat: 4 g, Carbohydrates: 18 g

Ingredients:
- 1 can (15 oz) chickpeas, drained and rinsed
- 1 tbsp olive oil
- 1 tsp paprika
- Salt to taste

Instructions:
- Preheat the oven to 400°F (200°C).
- Toss the chickpeas with olive oil, paprika, and salt.
- Spread the chickpeas on a baking sheet in a single layer.
- Roast for 25-30 minutes until crispy, shaking the pan halfway through.
- Let cool before serving.

Yogurt and Berry Smoothie

Serves: 1, Prep Time: 5 minutes, Total Time: 5 minutes

Calories: 150, Protein: 8 g, Fat: 2 g, Carbohydrates: 28 g

Ingredients:
- 1 cup Greek yogurt
- 1/2 cup mixed berries (fresh or frozen)
- 1/2 cup milk (dairy or non-dairy)
- 1 tbsp honey (optional)

Instructions:
- In a blender, combine Greek yogurt, mixed berries, milk, and honey.
- Blend until smooth.
- Serve immediately.

Pumpkin Seeds with Dried Cranberries

Serves: 2, Prep Time: 2 minutes, Total Time: 2 minutes

Calories: 200, Protein: 8 g, Fat: 12 g, Carbohydrates: 18 g

Ingredients:
- 1/2 cup roasted pumpkin seeds
- 1/4 cup dried cranberries

Instructions:
- Mix the pumpkin seeds and dried cranberries in a bowl.
- Serve as a crunchy and sweet snack.

Almond and Blueberry Energy Bites

**Serves: 12 bites, Prep Time: 10 minutes,
Total Time: 30 minutes (including refrigeration)**

Calories: 150, Protein: 4 g, Fat: 8 g, Carbohydrates: 18 g

Ingredients:
- 1 cup rolled oats
- 1/2 cup almond butter
- 1/4 cup honey
- 1/4 cup dried blueberries
- 1/4 cup chopped almonds

Instructions:
- In a large bowl, mix together rolled oats, almond butter, honey, dried blueberries, and chopped almonds.
- Form the mixture into small bites using your hands.
- Refrigerate for 20 minutes before serving.

CHAPTER 5
Delicious Calcium-Fortified Desserts

These calcium-fortified treats are not only delicious but also beneficial for maintaining strong bones.

Frozen Yogurt with Mixed Berries

- Serves: 4
- Prep Time: 5 minutes
- Cook Time: 20 minutes (churning)
- Total Time: 25 minutes

Nutrition per serving:
- Calories: 150
- Protein: 6 g
- Fat: 2 g
- Carbohydrates: 30 g

Ingredients:
- 2 cups plain Greek yogurt
- 1 cup mixed berries (strawberries, blueberries, raspberries)
- 2 tbsp honey
- 1 tsp vanilla extract

Instructions:
- Mix the Greek yogurt with honey and vanilla extract in a bowl.
- Pour the mixture into an ice cream maker and churn according to the manufacturer's instructions.
- Once frozen, fold in the mixed berries.
- Serve immediately or freeze for later.

Calcium-Fortified Rice Pudding

Serves: 4, Prep Time: 5 minutes, Cook Time: 30 minutes, Total Time: 35 minutes

Calories: 220, Protein: 6 g, Fat: 3 g, Carbohydrates: 40 g

Ingredients:
- 1/2 cup Arborio rice
- 2 cups calcium-fortified milk
- 1/4 cup sugar
- 1 tsp vanilla extract
- 1/4 tsp cinnamon
- 1/4 cup raisins (optional)

Instructions:
- In a medium saucepan, combine the rice, milk, and sugar.
- Cook over medium heat, stirring frequently, until the mixture thickens and the rice is tender, about 25-30 minutes.
- Stir in the vanilla extract, cinnamon, and raisins if using.
- Serve warm or chilled.

Almond and Dark Chocolate Bark

Serves: 8, Prep Time: 5 minutes, Cook Time: 5 minutes, Total Time: 40 minutes (including refrigeration)

Calories: 180, Protein: 3 g, Fat: 12 g, Carbohydrates: 18 g

Ingredients:
- 1 cup dark chocolate chips (70% cocoa or higher)
- 1/2 cup almonds, chopped
- 1/4 tsp sea salt

Instructions:
- Melt the dark chocolate chips in a double boiler or microwave, stirring until smooth.
- Spread the melted chocolate on a parchment-lined baking sheet in a thin layer.
- Sprinkle the chopped almonds and sea salt evenly over the chocolate.
- Refrigerate until the chocolate is set, about 30 minutes.
- Break into pieces and serve.

Orange and Yogurt Sorbet

Serves: 4, Prep Time: 5 minutes, Cook Time: 20 minutes (churning), Total Time: 25 minutes

Calories: 120, Protein: 3 g, Fat: 0 g, Carbohydrates: 25 g

Ingredients:

- 2 cups orange juice (freshly squeezed)
- 1 cup plain Greek yogurt
- 2 tbsp honey
- 1 tsp orange zest

Instructions:

- In a blender, combine the orange juice, Greek yogurt, honey, and orange zest.
- Blend until smooth.
- Pour the mixture into an ice cream maker and churn according to the manufacturer's instructions.
- Serve immediately or freeze for later.

Cheese and Fruit Platter

Serves: 2, Prep Time: 5 minutes, Total Time: 5 minutes

Calories: 200, Protein: 10 g, Fat: 12 g, Carbohydrates: 18 g

Ingredients:

- 2 oz assorted cheeses (cheddar, brie, gouda)
- 1 apple, sliced
- 1/4 cup grapes
- 1/4 cup dried apricots

Instructions:

- Arrange the cheese and fruit on a platter.
- Serve immediately.

Baked Apples with Cinnamon and Walnuts

Serves: 4, Prep Time: 10 minutes, Cook Time: 30 minutes, Total Time: 40 minutes

Calories: 180, Protein: 2 g, Fat: 6 g, Carbohydrates: 32 g

Ingredients:
- 4 apples, cored
- 1/4 cup walnuts, chopped
- 2 tbsp honey
- 1 tsp cinnamon
- 1 tbsp butter

Instructions:
- Preheat the oven to 350°F (175°C).
- In a small bowl, mix the walnuts, honey, and cinnamon.
- Stuff the mixture into the cored apples.
- Place the apples in a baking dish and top each with a small piece of butter.
- Bake for 25-30 minutes until the apples are tender.
- Serve warm.

Chia Pudding with Almond Milk and Fresh Berries

Serves: 2, Prep Time: 5 minutes, Total Time: 2 hours 5 minutes (including refrigeration)

Calories: 160, Protein: 4 g, Fat: 9 g, Carbohydrates: 18 g

Ingredients:
- 1/4 cup chia seeds
- 1 cup almond milk (calcium-fortified)
- 1 tbsp honey or maple syrup
- 1/2 cup mixed fresh berries

Instructions:
- In a bowl, combine chia seeds, almond milk, and honey or maple syrup.
- Stir well and refrigerate for at least 2 hours, or overnight, until the pudding thickens.
- Top with fresh berries before serving.

Greek Yogurt Cheesecake with Honey Drizzle

Serves: 8, Prep Time: 15 minutes, Cook Time: 35 minutes, Total Time: 50 minutes

Calories: 220, Protein: 8 g, Fat: 12 g, Carbohydrates: 24 g

Ingredients:
- 1 1/2 cups crushed graham crackers
- 1/4 cup melted butter
- 2 cups plain Greek yogurt
- 1/2 cup cream cheese
- 1/2 cup honey
- 1 tsp vanilla extract

Instructions:
- Preheat the oven to 325°F (160°C).
- Mix the crushed graham crackers with melted butter and press into the bottom of a springform pan.
- In a bowl, mix Greek yogurt, cream cheese, honey, and vanilla extract until smooth.
- Pour the mixture over the graham cracker crust.
- Bake for 30-35 minutes until set.
- Let cool, then drizzle with honey before serving.

Banana and Oat Cookies

Serves: 12 cookies, Prep Time: 10 minutes, Cook Time: 15

Calories: 100, Protein: 2 g, Fat: 3 g, Carbohydrates: 18 g

Ingredients:
- 2 ripe bananas, mashed
- 1 cup rolled oats
- 1/4 cup almond butter
- 1/4 cup dark chocolate chips (optional)

Instructions:
- Preheat the oven to 350°F (175°C).
- In a bowl, mix mashed bananas, rolled oats, almond butter, and chocolate chips if using.
- Drop spoonfuls of the mixture onto a baking sheet lined with parchment paper.
- Bake for 12-15 minutes until golden.
- Let cool before serving.

Calcium-Fortified Chocolate Pudding

**Serves: 4, Prep Time: 5 minutes, Cook Time: 10 minutes,
Total Time: 1 hour 15 minutes (including refrigeration)**

Calories: 190, Protein: 6 g, Fat: 6 g, Carbohydrates: 30 g

Ingredients:
- 2 cups calcium-fortified milk
- 1/4 cup cocoa powder
- 1/4 cup sugar
- 3 tbsp cornstarch
- 1/4 tsp vanilla extract
- Pinch of salt

Instructions:
- In a medium saucepan, whisk together cocoa powder, sugar, cornstarch, and salt.
- Slowly add the calcium-fortified milk, whisking constantly to avoid lumps.
- Cook over medium heat, stirring constantly, until the mixture thickens (about 5-7 minutes).
- Remove from heat and stir in the vanilla extract.
- Pour into serving bowls and refrigerate for at least 1 hour before serving.

Strawberry and Yogurt Popsicles

**Serves: 6 popsicles, Prep Time: 5 minutes,
Total Time: 4 hours 5 minutes (including freezing)**

Calories: 80, Protein: 3 g, Fat: 1 g, Carbohydrates: 15 g

Ingredients:
- 1 cup plain Greek yogurt
- 1/2 cup strawberries, chopped
- 1 tbsp honey
- 1/4 cup calcium-fortified orange juice

Instructions:
- In a blender, combine Greek yogurt, strawberries, honey, and orange juice.
- Blend until smooth.
- Pour the mixture into popsicle molds and freeze for at least 4 hours or until solid.
- Serve immediately.

Blueberry and Almond Milk Smoothie Bowl

Serves: 1, Prep Time: 5 minutes, Total Time: 5 minutes

Calories: 220, Protein: 6 g, Fat: 8 g, Carbohydrates: 30 g

Ingredients:
- 1/2 cup frozen blueberries
- 1/2 cup calcium-fortified almond milk
- 1 tbsp almond butter
- 1/4 cup granola
- 1 tbsp chia seeds
- Fresh blueberries for topping

Instructions:
- Blend the frozen blueberries, almond milk, and almond butter until smooth.
- Pour into a bowl and top with granola, chia seeds, and fresh blueberries.
- Serve immediately.

Apricot and Almond Energy Bars

**Serves: 8 bars, Prep Time: 10 minutes,
Total Time: 2 hours 10 minutes (including refrigeration)**

Calories: 150, Protein: 4 g, Fat: 7 g, Carbohydrates: 18 g

Ingredients:
- 1 cup dried apricots
- 1/2 cup almonds, chopped
- 1 cup rolled oats
- 1/4 cup honey
- 1/4 cup almond butter

Instructions:
- In a food processor, pulse the dried apricots and almonds until finely chopped.
- In a bowl, combine the oats, honey, almond butter, and apricot-almond mixture.
- Press the mixture into an 8x8-inch baking dish.
- Refrigerate for 2 hours, then cut into bars.
- Store in an airtight container.

Peach and Greek Yogurt Crumble

Serves: 4, Prep Time: 10 minutes, Cook Time: 20 minutes, Total Time: 30 minutes

Calories: 180, Protein: 6 g, Fat: 5 g, Carbohydrates: 30 g

Ingredients:
- 4 ripe peaches, sliced
- 1/2 cup plain Greek yogurt
- 1/4 cup rolled oats
- 1 tbsp honey
- 2 tbsp almond flour
- 1/4 tsp cinnamon

Instructions:
- Preheat the oven to 350°F (175°C).
- Arrange the peach slices in a baking dish.
- In a small bowl, mix the oats, almond flour, cinnamon, and honey.
- Sprinkle the mixture over the peaches.
- Bake for 20 minutes, until the topping is golden and the peaches are tender.
- Serve with a dollop of Greek yogurt.

Baked Pears with Ricotta and Honey

Serves: 4, Prep Time: 5 minutes, Cook Time: 25 minutes, Total Time: 30 minutes

Calories: 150, Protein: 5 g, Fat: 5 g, Carbohydrates: 25 g

Ingredients:
- 2 pears, halved and cored
- 1/4 cup ricotta cheese
- 2 tbsp honey
- 1/4 tsp cinnamon

Instructions:
- Preheat the oven to 350°F (175°C).
- Place the pear halves in a baking dish.
- Spoon ricotta cheese into the center of each pear half.
- Drizzle with honey and sprinkle with cinnamon.
- Bake for 20-25 minutes until the pears are soft.
- Serve warm.

CHAPTER 6
Magnesium-Powered Meals

Magnesium plays a critical role in maintaining bone density by helping the body properly absorb calcium. A deficiency in magnesium can lead to bone loss, making it a key nutrient for seniors managing osteoporosis. Magnesium works hand-in-hand with calcium to strengthen bones, ensuring that calcium is properly utilized for bone repair and growth.

Quinoa and Avocado Salad with Pumpkin Seeds

Serves: 2, Prep Time: 10 minutes, Total Time: 10 minutes

Calories: 300, Protein: 8 g, Fat: 18 g, Carbohydrates: 26 g

Ingredients:
- 1 cup cooked quinoa
- 1 ripe avocado, sliced
- 1/4 cup pumpkin seeds
- 1/4 cup cherry tomatoes, halved
- 1 tbsp olive oil
- Juice of 1 lime
- Salt and pepper to taste

Instructions:
- In a bowl, combine cooked quinoa, sliced avocado, pumpkin seeds, and cherry tomatoes.
- Drizzle with olive oil and lime juice, and season with salt and pepper.
- Toss everything together and serve chilled or at room temperature.

Roasted Salmon with Spinach and Almonds

Serves: 2, Prep Time: 5 minutes, Cook Time: 15 minutes, Total Time: 20 minutes

Nutrition per serving:
- Calories: 400
- Protein: 30 g
- Fat: 25 g
- Carbohydrates: 10 g

Ingredients:
- 2 salmon fillets
- 2 cups fresh spinach
- 1/4 cup sliced almonds
- 1 tbsp olive oil
- 1 garlic clove, minced
- Salt and pepper to taste

Instructions:
- Preheat oven to 375°F (190°C).
- Place salmon fillets on a baking sheet, drizzle with olive oil, and season with salt and pepper.
- Roast for 15 minutes or until the salmon flakes easily with a fork.
- While the salmon is roasting, sauté spinach in a pan with garlic and a little olive oil until wilted.
- Sprinkle with almonds and serve with roasted salmon.

Lentil and Kale Soup

Serves: 4, Prep Time: 10 minutes, Cook Time: 30 minutes, Total Time: 40 minutes

- **Nutrition per serving:**
- Calories: 250
- Protein: 12 g
- Fat: 4 g
- Carbohydrates: 42 g

Ingredients:
- 1 cup dried lentils, rinsed
- 2 cups kale, chopped
- 1 onion, diced
- 2 garlic cloves, minced
- 1 carrot, diced
- 1 celery stalk, diced
- 4 cups vegetable broth
- 1 tsp cumin
- Salt and pepper to taste

Instructions:
- In a large pot, sauté onion, garlic, carrot, and celery until soft.
- Add lentils, vegetable broth, and cumin.
- Bring to a boil, then reduce heat and simmer for 25 minutes or until lentils are tender.
- Stir in chopped kale and cook for an additional 5 minutes.
- Season with salt and pepper, then serve hot.

Grilled Chicken with Swiss Chard and Brown Rice

Serves: 2, Prep Time: 10 minutes, Cook Time: 15 minutes, Total Time: 25 minutes

Calories: 350, Protein: 30 g, Fat: 10 g, Carbohydrates: 35 g

Ingredients:
- 2 boneless, skinless chicken breasts
- 2 cups Swiss chard, chopped
- 1 cup cooked brown rice
- 1 tbsp olive oil
- Salt and pepper to taste

Instructions:
- Season chicken breasts with salt and pepper and grill for 6-8 minutes on each side, or until fully cooked.
- In a pan, sauté Swiss chard in olive oil until wilted.
- Serve the grilled chicken over brown rice, with sautéed Swiss chard on the side.

Baked Sweet Potatoes with Greek Yogurt and Pumpkin Seeds

Serves: 2, Prep Time: 5 minutes, Cook Time: 45 minutes, Total Time: 50 minutes

Calories: 280, Protein: 8 g, Fat: 10 g, Carbohydrates: 40 g

Ingredients:
- 2 medium sweet potatoes
- 1/2 cup Greek yogurt
- 2 tbsp pumpkin seeds
- 1 tbsp honey (optional)
- Salt and pepper to taste

Instructions:
- Preheat oven to 375°F (190°C).
- Pierce the sweet potatoes with a fork and bake for 45 minutes or until tender.
- Once baked, slice the sweet potatoes open and top with Greek yogurt, pumpkin seeds, and a drizzle of honey if desired.
- Season with a pinch of salt and pepper before serving.

Tofu Stir-Fry with Broccoli and Cashews

Serves: 2, Prep Time: 10 minutes, Cook Time: 10 minutes, Total Time: 20 minutes

- **Nutrition per serving:**
- Calories: 300
- Protein: 15 g
- Fat: 15 g
- Carbohydrates: 25 g

Ingredients:

- 1 block firm tofu, cubed
- 2 cups broccoli florets
- 1/4 cup cashews
- 2 tbsp soy sauce
- 1 tbsp sesame oil
- 1 garlic clove, minced
- 1 tsp ginger, minced

Instructions:

- In a pan, heat sesame oil and sauté tofu until golden on all sides.
- Add garlic, ginger, and broccoli, stir-frying for about 5 minutes until tender.
- Stir in soy sauce and cashews, and cook for another 2 minutes.
- Serve hot with rice or quinoa.

Sweet Potato and Black Bean Tacos

Serves: 4 (2 tacos each), Prep Time: 10 minutes, Cook Time: 25 minutes, Total Time: 35 minutes

- **Nutrition per serving:**
- Calories: 320
- Protein: 9 g
- Fat: 8 g
- Carbohydrates: 55 g

Ingredients:
- 2 medium sweet potatoes, diced
- 1 can (15 oz) black beans, drained and rinsed
- 8 small corn tortillas
- 1/4 cup cilantro, chopped
- 1/2 cup red onion, diced
- 1 tsp cumin
- 1 tbsp olive oil
- Juice of 1 lime
- Salt and pepper to taste

Instructions:
- Preheat oven to 400°F (200°C).
- Toss sweet potatoes with olive oil, cumin, salt, and pepper. Spread them on a baking sheet and roast for 25 minutes or until tender.
- Heat black beans in a small pot.
- Warm the tortillas and assemble tacos by layering black beans, roasted sweet potatoes, red onion, and cilantro. Squeeze lime juice over the top before serving.

Spinach and Mushroom Frittata with Feta

Serves: 4, Prep Time: 10 minutes, Cook Time: 15 minutes, Total Time: 25 minutes

- **Nutrition per serving:**
- Calories: 280
- Protein: 15 g
- Fat: 18 g
- Carbohydrates: 10 g

Ingredients:
- 6 large eggs
- 2 cups fresh spinach, chopped
- 1 cup mushrooms, sliced
- 1/4 cup feta cheese, crumbled
- 1 tbsp olive oil
- Salt and pepper to taste

Instructions:
- Preheat oven to 350°F (175°C).
- Heat olive oil in an oven-safe skillet and sauté mushrooms until browned. Add spinach and cook until wilted.
- In a bowl, whisk the eggs, then pour them over the vegetables in the skillet. Sprinkle feta on top.
- Cook on the stovetop for 2-3 minutes until the edges set, then transfer to the oven and bake for 10-12 minutes, or until the frittata is fully cooked through.
- Slice and serve warm.

Chickpea and Spinach Curry

Serves: 4, Prep Time: 10 minutes, Cook Time: 20 minutes, Total Time: 30 minutes

- **Nutrition per serving:**
- Calories: 320
- Protein: 10 g
- Fat: 14 g
- Carbohydrates: 40 g

Ingredients:
- 1 can (15 oz) chickpeas, drained and rinsed
- 2 cups fresh spinach, chopped
- 1 onion, diced
- 2 garlic cloves, minced
- 1 tbsp curry powder
- 1 can (14 oz) diced tomatoes
- 1/2 cup coconut milk
- 1 tbsp olive oil
- Salt and pepper to taste

Instructions:
- Heat olive oil in a pan and sauté onion and garlic until soft.
- Add curry powder and cook for 1 minute.
- Stir in chickpeas, diced tomatoes, and coconut milk. Simmer for 15 minutes.
- Add spinach and cook for another 5 minutes until wilted. Season with salt and pepper.
- Serve over rice or with whole grain naan.

Baked Cod with Quinoa and Wilted Kale

Serves: 2, Prep Time: 10 minutes, Cook Time: 15 minutes, Total Time: 25 minutes

Calories: 340, Protein: 28 g, Fat: 10 g, Carbohydrates: 35 g

Ingredients:
- 2 cod fillets
- 1 cup cooked quinoa
- 2 cups kale, chopped
- 1 tbsp olive oil
- 1 lemon, sliced
- Salt and pepper to taste

Instructions:
- Preheat oven to 375°F (190°C).
- Place cod fillets on a baking sheet, drizzle with olive oil, and season with salt, pepper, and lemon slices. Bake for 12-15 minutes or until the fish flakes easily.
- In a skillet, sauté kale in a bit of olive oil until wilted.
- Serve the baked cod over quinoa with the wilted kale on the side.

Roasted Turkey with Garlic Mashed Sweet Potatoes

Serves: 2, Prep Time: 10 minutes, Cook Time: 30 minutes, Total Time: 40 minutes

Calories: 380, Protein: 28 g, Fat: 12 g, Carbohydrates: 45 g

Ingredients:
- 2 turkey breasts
- 2 medium sweet potatoes, peeled and chopped
- 2 garlic cloves, minced
- 1 tbsp olive oil
- 1/4 cup low-fat milk
- Salt and pepper to taste

Instructions:
- Preheat oven to 375°F (190°C). Season turkey breasts with salt and pepper, and roast for 25-30 minutes or until fully cooked.
- Meanwhile, boil sweet potatoes until tender. Drain, and mash with garlic, olive oil, and milk until smooth. Season with salt and pepper.
- Serve roasted turkey with garlic mashed sweet potatoes.

Shrimp and Spinach Sauté with Almonds

Serves: 2, Prep Time: 10 minutes, Cook Time: 10 minutes, Total Time: 20 minutes

- **Nutrition per serving:**
- Calories: 320
- Protein: 25 g
- Fat: 18 g
- Carbohydrates: 10 g

Ingredients:
- 1 lb shrimp, peeled and deveined
- 2 cups spinach, chopped
- 1/4 cup sliced almonds
- 1 tbsp olive oil
- 2 garlic cloves, minced
- Juice of 1 lemon
- Salt and pepper to taste

Instructions:
- Heat olive oil in a large pan and sauté garlic until fragrant.
- Add shrimp and cook for 3-4 minutes until they turn pink.
- Stir in spinach and cook until wilted, about 2 minutes.
- Sprinkle almonds on top, season with salt, pepper, and lemon juice.
- Serve hot with your choice of whole grains or quinoa.

Grilled Tofu with Stir-Fried Bok Choy and Sesame Seeds

Serves: 2, Prep Time: 10 minutes, Cook Time: 10 minutes, Total Time: 20 minutes

- **Nutrition per serving:**
- Calories: 280
- Protein: 15 g
- Fat: 15 g
- Carbohydrates: 20 g

Ingredients:
- 1 block firm tofu, pressed and sliced
- 2 cups bok choy, chopped
- 1 tbsp sesame oil
- 1 tbsp soy sauce
- 1 tsp sesame seeds
- 1 garlic clove, minced
- Salt and pepper to taste

Instructions:
- Grill the tofu slices on both sides for 5-6 minutes or until browned.
- In a pan, heat sesame oil and sauté garlic until fragrant. Add bok choy and cook until tender, about 5 minutes.
- Stir in soy sauce and sesame seeds.
- Serve the grilled tofu over the bok choy mixture.

Lentil and Quinoa Stuffed Bell Peppers

Serves: 4, Prep Time: 15 minutes, Cook Time: 25 minutes, Total Time: 40 minutes

- **Nutrition per serving:**
- Calories: 350
- Protein: 15 g
- Fat: 8 g
- Carbohydrates: 55 g

Ingredients:
- 4 large bell peppers, tops cut off and seeds removed
- 1 cup cooked lentils
- 1/2 cup cooked quinoa
- 1/2 cup diced tomatoes
- 1 onion, diced
- 1 tbsp olive oil
- 1 tsp cumin
- Salt and pepper to taste

Instructions:
- Preheat oven to 375°F (190°C).
- Sauté onion in olive oil until soft. Add lentils, quinoa, diced tomatoes, and cumin. Cook for 5 minutes.
- Stuff the bell peppers with the lentil-quinoa mixture and place them in a baking dish.
- Bake for 25 minutes until the peppers are tender.
- Serve hot.

Turkey Meatballs with Spinach and Chickpeas

Serves: 4, Prep Time: 15 minutes, Cook Time: 25 minutes, Total Time: 40 minutes

- **Nutrition per serving:**
- Calories: 380
- Protein: 25 g
- Fat: 15 g
- Carbohydrates: 35 g

Ingredients:
- 1 lb ground turkey
- 1 cup spinach, chopped
- 1/2 cup cooked chickpeas, mashed
- 1 egg
- 1/4 cup breadcrumbs
- 2 garlic cloves, minced
- 1 tbsp olive oil
- Salt and pepper to taste

Instructions:
- Preheat oven to 375°F (190°C).
- In a bowl, mix ground turkey, spinach, chickpeas, egg, breadcrumbs, garlic, salt, and pepper.
- Shape the mixture into small meatballs and place them on a baking sheet.
- Bake for 20-25 minutes until fully cooked.
- Serve with your choice of vegetables or whole grain pasta.

Roasted Cauliflower with Tahini and Pine Nuts

Serves: 4, Prep Time: 10 minutes, Cook Time: 25 minutes, Total Time: 35 minutes

- **Nutrition per serving:**
- Calories: 260
- Protein: 8 g
- Fat: 18 g
- Carbohydrates: 18 g

Ingredients:
- 1 head cauliflower, chopped into florets
- 2 tbsp tahini
- 1 tbsp olive oil
- 2 tbsp lemon juice
- 1/4 cup pine nuts
- Salt and pepper to taste

Instructions:
- Preheat oven to 400°F (200°C).
- Toss cauliflower florets with olive oil, salt, and pepper, and spread on a baking sheet.
- Roast for 25 minutes or until golden and tender.
- Drizzle tahini and lemon juice over the roasted cauliflower and sprinkle with pine nuts.
- Serve hot.

CHAPTER 7
Meal Planning and Prep Tips for Seniors

Eating well is crucial for managing osteoporosis, but preparing healthy meals can be challenging for seniors, especially when time, energy, and resources are limited. This chapter will simplify meal prep, offer budget-friendly shopping tips, and provide practical advice for seniors or caregivers preparing meals.

Simplifying Meal Preparation
- Focus on recipes with minimal ingredients and simple techniques.
- Use batch cooking to save time.
- Incorporate one-pan meals to reduce cleanup.
- Prioritize nutrient-dense, bone-healthy foods in every meal.

Budget-Friendly Shopping Tips for Bone-Healthy Foods
- Buy in bulk: Purchase long-lasting items like beans, whole grains, and nuts.
- Opt for frozen vegetables and fruits, which are often cheaper and just as nutritious as fresh produce.
- Shop seasonally to take advantage of fresh, affordable produce.
- Look for sales and coupons on calcium-fortified foods like dairy or plant-based alternatives.

Grocery Shopping List for Bone Health
A basic shopping list to make sure you have all the essential ingredients for bone-strengthening meals:

- Proteins: Eggs, lean chicken, turkey, salmon, sardines, tofu, beans, lentils.
- Dairy/Alternatives: Greek yogurt, cottage cheese, fortified plant-based milk, ricotta.
- Fruits: Berries, bananas, apples, oranges.
- Vegetables: Spinach, kale, broccoli, sweet potatoes, mushrooms.
- Grains: Quinoa, brown rice, whole grain bread, oats.
- Nuts/Seeds: Almonds, chia seeds, sunflower seeds, pumpkin seeds.
- Fortified Foods: Calcium-fortified cereal, fortified orange juice.

Tips for Cooking for One or Two
- Use portioned ingredients to prevent food waste.
- Invest in single-serve containers for meal prepping.
- Create versatile dishes (like soups or casseroles) that can be eaten over multiple days.
- Freeze leftovers in single portions for quick reheating.

How to Freeze Meals for Future Use
- Freeze food in portion sizes for easy reheating.
- Label containers with the date and meal type to prevent confusion.
- Cool dishes completely before freezing to preserve quality.
- Avoid freezing foods like lettuce or cucumbers, which don't freeze well.

Quick and Nutritious Lunch Box Ideas
- Prepare wraps with turkey, avocado, and spinach.
- Pack salads that include quinoa, nuts, and protein like grilled chicken.
- Create snack packs with cheese, whole grain crackers, and fruit.
- Opt for bento boxes with a balance of protein, healthy fats, and whole grains.

Building Balanced Meals with Calcium and Vitamin D
- Combine dairy or fortified plant-based alternatives with leafy greens.
- Pair calcium-rich meals with foods high in vitamin D, like fatty fish or fortified cereals.
- Include a source of healthy fats (avocado, olive oil) to enhance nutrient absorption.

Using Leftovers Creatively
- Use leftover vegetables to make soups or stir-fries.
- Add extra cooked chicken or tofu to salads or wraps for a quick lunch.
- Incorporate leftover grains like quinoa into breakfast bowls with nuts.

Portion Control for Seniors
- Use smaller plates to avoid overeating.
- Measure ingredients for accuracy, especially for calorie-dense foods like nuts
- Divide meals into multiple smaller servings to be eaten throughout the day.

Incorporating Seasonal Produce
- In summer, choose fresh berries, tomatoes, and leafy greens.
- In fall and winter, focus on root vegetables like sweet potatoes and squash.
- Purchase local produce when it's in season for both freshness and affordability

Meal Prep Tips for Busy Days
- Designate one day a week for meal prep and cooking.
- Utilize slow cookers or instant pots for hands-off cooking.
- Prep ingredients in advance (chop vegetables, cook grains) to make assembly easier during the week.

Cooking on a Budget
- Purchase generic brands, which are often cheaper but just as nutritious.
- Plan meals around sales and discounts at the grocery store.
- Use beans, lentils, and grains as budget-friendly alternatives to animal protein.

Smart Storage Solutions for Fresh Ingredients
- Store fresh herbs in water to prolong their shelf life.
- Keep leafy greens wrapped in a damp towel in the fridge.
- Use airtight containers to store dry goods and prevent spoilage.

Minimizing Food Waste
- Plan meals around perishable ingredients to use them before they spoil.
- Repurpose ingredients (e.g., roasted vegetables for soups, or grain leftovers in salads).
- Freeze produce that you won't use immediately to extend its life.

Easy-to-Cook Recipes for Caregivers
- Focus on one-pot or one-pan meals that require minimal prep and cleanup.
- Create a recipe rotation of quick meals (e.g., grilled chicken with vegetables, stir-fries).
- Batch-cook and freeze meals that can be quickly reheated, like soups, stews, and casseroles

Exercise Tips to Prevent Bone Loss

1. Weight-Bearing Exercises
Walking: A low-impact activity that strengthens bones in the legs, hips, and lower spine. It's also advisable to aim for at least 30 minutes most days of the week.
Dancing: Fun and effective for improving bone density in the lower body. You can join a dance class or dance at home to your favorite music.
Hiking: Provides a challenging, varied terrain that enhances bone strength. You can start with easy trails and then, gradually progress to more challenging ones.

2. Resistance Training
Bodyweight Exercises: Push-ups, squats, and lunges use your own body weight to build strength. You can start with lower repetitions and then, gradually increase as you build strength.
Resistance Bands: These offer adjustable resistance and are great for exercises like bicep curls, leg lifts, and shoulder presses.
Free Weights: Use dumbbells or kettlebells for exercises such as deadlifts, bench presses, and rows. Focus on proper form and start with lighter weights.

3. Balance and Flexibility Exercises
Tai Chi: This ancient practice improves balance, flexibility, and coordination, reducing the risk of falls and fractures.
Yoga: Gentle stretching and strengthening exercises help maintain flexibility and bone strength. Poses like Tree Pose, Warrior Pose, and Bridge Pose are particularly beneficial.
Balance Exercises: Stand on one leg, or use a balance board to enhance stability. This helps in preventing falls and strengthening core muscles.

4. High-Impact Exercises (For Those with Osteoporosis Approval)
Jumping: If advised by your healthcare provider, low-impact jumping exercises like jumping jacks or skipping rope can help improve bone density.
Stair Climbing: Climbing stairs provides weight-bearing activity that strengthens bones. Use a stairwell or stair machine at the gym.

5. Low-Impact Exercises
Swimming: This could provide a full-body workout without putting stress on the joints. Great for overall fitness and bone health.
Cycling: Builds muscle and endurance without high-impact stress on the bones. Use a stationary bike for indoor exercise.

6. Safe Exercise Practices
Warm-Up and Cool Down: Always start with a warm-up to prepare your muscles and bones for exercise, and finish with a cool-down to prevent stiffness and injury.
Proper Technique: It's important to use correct form and technique to avoid injury. Consider working with a trainer or physical therapist to ensure proper execution.

CHAPTER 8
Staying Active and Hydrated

The Importance of Exercise in Supporting Bone Health
Exercise is essential for keeping bones strong and healthy. Engaging in regular physical activity, especially weight-bearing exercises, helps to slow down bone loss and even strengthen bones. Exercise also improves balance and coordination, which reduces the risk of falls—a major concern for people with osteoporosis.

Hydration Tips for Seniors
Staying hydrated is important for overall health, but it becomes even more critical as we age. Proper hydration helps maintain joint function, supports digestion, and keeps our body functioning properly. Sometimes, we may not feel as thirsty as we did when we were younger, so it's important to consciously drink water throughout the day.

Lifestyle Tips:
- **Low-Impact Exercises for Bone Strength:** Low-impact exercises are gentle on the joints but still strengthen bones. Activities like walking, swimming, and cycling can help you stay fit without putting too much pressure on your knees or hips. Chair exercises or using resistance bands are also great options to build strength while seated or standing.

- **Incorporating Hydration into Daily Routine:** Make drinking water a habit. You can start your day with a glass of water and drink small amounts regularly throughout the day. Setting reminders on your phone or placing water bottles around the house can help you remember to sip regularly.

- **Combining Diet and Exercise for Optimal Results:** Eating bone-healthy foods and exercising regularly is the best combination for maintaining strong bones. For example, eating calcium-rich foods like yogurt or spinach before a workout provides the nutrients your body needs to strengthen bones during physical activity.

- **Simple Stretching Routines for Seniors:** Gentle stretches help improve flexibility and mobility, which are important for maintaining good posture and reducing stiffness. You can start by stretching your arms, legs, and back each morning to keep your body limber. Stretching while seated or holding onto a sturdy chair can help with balance.

- **Water-Rich Foods to Boost Hydration:** Eating foods that have a high water content is a great way to stay hydrated without having to drink more water. Examples of water-rich foods include cucumbers, watermelon, oranges, and leafy greens. Adding these to your meals helps ensure you stay hydrated throughout the day.

- **Bone-Strengthening Exercises to Try at Home:** You don't need fancy equipment to do exercises that strengthen your bones. Simple activities like standing on one leg to improve balance, lifting light hand weights, or doing wall push-ups can be done at home. These exercises help build muscle and protect your bones from breaking.

- **Staying Hydrated with Herbal Teas:** If plain water gets boring, try drinking herbal teas. They can be a great alternative to sugary drinks, and many herbal teas have additional benefits like soothing the digestive system. Opt for decaffeinated teas to avoid dehydration.

- **Daily Walking for Improved Mobility:** Walking is one of the best exercises for seniors. It's gentle on the joints, doesn't require any special equipment, and helps improve bone density. Aim for a short walk every day, even if it's just around the block or inside the house. Walking also improves balance and boosts overall well-being.

- **Yoga Poses for Bone Health:** Yoga helps improve flexibility, balance, and strength. Certain yoga poses, like the tree pose or warrior pose, are especially good for building strength in the legs and hips. These poses are gentle and can be adapted to suit different ability levels. Yoga also helps with relaxation, which is important for mental well-being.

- **Hydration Tips for Warmer Weather:** In hot weather, it's easy to become dehydrated without realizing it. Make sure you're drinking water regularly, even if you're not thirsty. Keep a bottle of water with you when you're outside or doing any physical activities. You can also eat hydrating snacks like watermelon or cold cucumber slices to help stay cool.

- **Balancing Exercise and Rest:** It's important to strike a balance between staying active and allowing your body time to rest. If you feel tired or sore, listen to your body and take a break. Regular rest helps your muscles recover and prevents injury. Aim for a mix of activity and relaxation every day.

- **Monitoring Bone Health with Regular Check-Ups:** Staying on top of your bone health is important, especially as you age. Make sure to visit your healthcare provider for regular check-ups and bone density scans. These tests help monitor your bone health and ensure that you're doing everything you can to protect your bones.

- **Hydration Tips for Cold Weather:** In colder weather, it's common to feel less thirsty, but your body still needs hydration. Warm drinks like herbal teas or soups can help keep you hydrated. You can also eat fruits like oranges and apples, which are hydrating and full of nutrients to boost your immune system.

- **Importance of Posture in Bone Health** Good posture is essential for keeping your spine healthy and reducing the risk of back pain or injury. Practice sitting and standing up straight, keeping your shoulders back and head held high. This also strengthens your core muscles, which support your spine.

- **Using Resistance Bands for Strength Training** Resistance bands are easy-to-use tools that help build strength without putting too much strain on your joints. You can use them to exercise your arms, legs, and core muscles. I will advice that you start with light resistance and then, gradually increase as your strength improves.

- **Creating a Daily Exercise Routine** Sticking to a daily exercise routine helps make physical activity a habit. Start with 10-15 minutes of activity per day and slowly increase the duration as you feel stronger. Including a variety of exercises—like walking, stretching, and strength training—ensures you're working different muscle groups while protecting your bones.

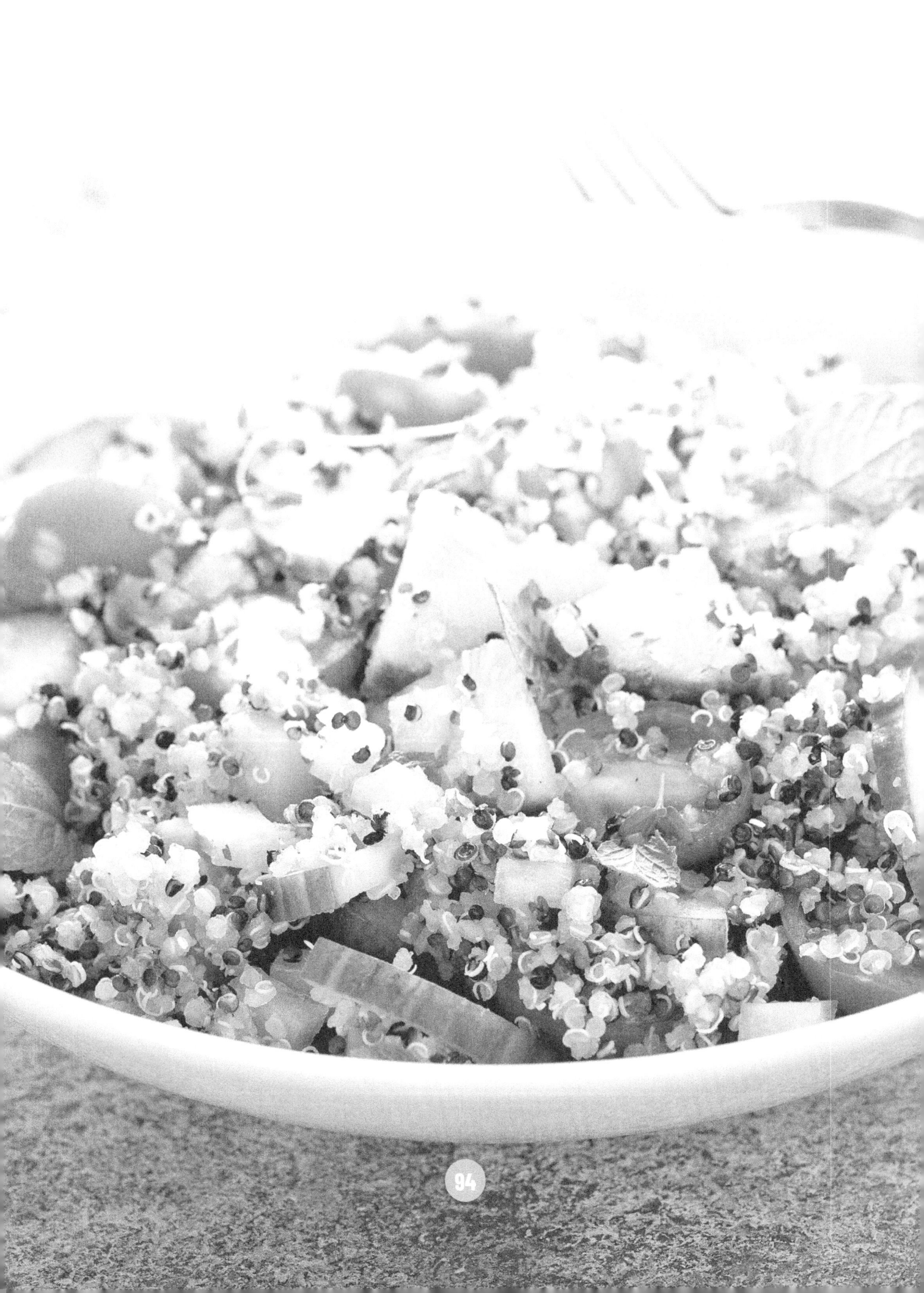

CONCLUSION

As you've journeyed through the pages of "Osteoporosis Diet Cookbook for Seniors," I hope you've discovered more than just recipes—I hope you've found a renewed sense of confidence in your ability to care for your bones, your health, and your future.

Osteoporosis may present challenges, but with the right knowledge, tools, and diet, it's a condition you can manage. The meals, tips, and strategies shared in this book are designed to fit easily into your lifestyle, providing nourishment and joy to each meal.

Remember, taking control of your bone health doesn't require complicated routines or bland food. it's as simple as enjoying the nutritious and delicious meals you've learned to prepare here.

As you move forward, keep in mind that every bite you take is a step toward stronger bones and a healthier, more vibrant life. The journey to better bone health isn't a sprint but a lifelong commitment, and you are already on the right path.

My hope is that this cookbook becomes a staple in your kitchen, a companion in your journey to wellness, and a reminder that it's never too late to invest in your health.

Wishing you strength, health, and happiness. one meal at a time.

A Heartfelt Thank You: Your Journey with This Cookbook

Dear Cherished Reader,

From the bottom of my heart, I want to extend my deepest gratitude for choosing this cookbook to support your health journey. Each recipe within these pages was created with care and compassion, with the hope of making your path to stronger bones and better well-being just a little bit easier.

Knowing that these meals have been a part of your daily routine fills me with profound joy. Your health, comfort, and happiness mean everything to me, and it's an honor to have contributed, even in a small way, to your journey toward better health.

As an independent author, your feedback isn't just important—it's the heartbeat of my work. If this cookbook has brought you hope, healing, or simply a little more joy in the kitchen, I would be so touched if you could take a moment to share your experience in a review on Amazon. Your words have the power to uplift others who, like you, are seeking a gentle hand of guidance toward a healthier life.

Your support fuels my passion and strengthens my resolve to continue creating resources that make a real difference in the lives of seniors striving for strength and vitality. I truly couldn't do it without you.

With all my appreciation and love

Ovia Cooper

BONUS WEEK ONE MEAL PLAN

MONDAY	**Day 1:** • Breakfast: Creamy Greek Yogurt Parfait with Berries and Nuts • Lunch: Grilled Salmon Salad with Citrus Vinaigrette • Dinner: Roasted Chicken with Quinoa and Steamed Broccoli • Snack/Dessert: Frozen Yogurt with Mixed Berries
TUESDAY	**Day 2:** • Breakfast: Spinach and Cheese Omelette • Lunch: Mushroom and Tofu Stir-Fry • Dinner: Lentil and Vegetable Stew • Snack/Dessert: Roasted Almonds and Dried Fruit Mix
WEDNESDAY	**Day 3:** • Breakfast: Almond Milk and Chia Seed Pudding • Lunch: Turkey and Avocado Wrap with Spinach • Dinner: Grilled Tofu with Stir-Fried Vegetables • Snack/Dessert: Greek Yogurt with Honey and Granola
THURSDAY	**Day 4:** • Breakfast: Whole Grain Cereal with Fortified Milk • Lunch: Sardine and Tomato Whole Grain Sandwich • Dinner: Baked Cod with Sweet Potato and Asparagus • Snack/Dessert: Pumpkin Seeds with Dried Cranberries
FRIDAY	**Day 5:** • Breakfast: Baked Oatmeal with Apples and Walnuts • Lunch: Quinoa Salad with Kale and Grilled Chicken • Dinner: Beef and Vegetable Stir-Fry with Brown Rice • Snack/Dessert: Almond and Blueberry Energy Bites
SATURDAY	**Day 6:** • Breakfast: Ricotta and Honey on Whole Grain Toast • Lunch: Egg Salad with Fresh Herbs • Dinner: Stuffed Bell Peppers with Quinoa and Ground Turkey • Snack/Dessert: Baked Apples with Cinnamon and Walnuts
SUNDAY	**Day 7:** • Breakfast: Smoothie with Kale, Almond Butter, and Fortified Orange Juice • Lunch: Tuna Salad with Lemon and Dill • Dinner: Grilled Shrimp Skewers with Veggie Couscous • Snack/Dessert: Chia Pudding with Almond Milk and Fresh Berries

BONUS WEEK TWO MEAL PLAN

MONDAY	**Day 8:** • Breakfast: Scrambled Eggs with Spinach and Feta • Lunch: Vitamin D-Fortified Soup with Chicken and Vegetables • Dinner: Vegetarian Chili with Black Beans and Sweet Corn • Snack/Dessert: Cheese and Whole Grain Crackers
TUESDAY	**Day 9:** • Breakfast: Overnight Oats with Chia Seeds and Almonds • Lunch: Shrimp and Avocado Salad • Dinner: Herb-Crusted Pork Tenderloin with Roasted Root Vegetables • Snack/Dessert: Calcium-Fortified Chocolate Pudding
WEDNESDAY	**Day 10:** • Breakfast: Quinoa Breakfast Bowl with Blueberries and Almonds • Lunch: Spinach and Mushroom Frittata • Dinner: Mushroom Risotto with Parmesan • Snack/Dessert: Roasted Chickpeas with Paprika
THURSDAY	**Day 11:** • Breakfast: Calcium-Fortified Pancakes with Maple Syrup • Lunch: Grilled Portobello Mushrooms with Quinoa • Dinner: Spaghetti with Turkey Meatballs and Marinara Sauce • Snack/Dessert: Strawberry and Yogurt Popsicles
FRIDAY	**Day 12:** • Breakfast: Cottage Cheese with Pineapple and Walnuts • Lunch: Chickpea and Spinach Salad with Sunflower Seeds • Dinner: Salmon with Wild Rice and Green Beans • Snack/Dessert: Dark Chocolate-Covered Almonds
SATURDAY	**Day 13:** • Breakfast: Tofu Scramble with Vegetables • Lunch: Smoked Salmon and Cucumber Sandwich • Dinner: Baked Eggplant Parmesan with Whole Grain Pasta • Snack/Dessert: Peach and Greek Yogurt Crumble
SUNDAY	**Day 14:** • Breakfast: Calcium-Fortified Waffles with Berry Compote • Lunch: Roasted Veggie and Tofu Bowl • Dinner: Chicken and Broccoli Stir-Fry with Brown Rice • Snack/Dessert: Yogurt and Berry Smoothie

BONUS WEEK THREE MEAL PLAN

MONDAY	**Day 15:** • <u>Breakfast:</u> Baked Egg Cups with Cheese and Spinach • <u>Lunch:</u> Grilled Tilapia with Steamed Broccoli • <u>Dinner:</u> Quinoa-Stuffed Zucchini Boats • <u>Snack/Dessert:</u> Calcium-Fortified Rice Pudding
TUESDAY	**Day 16:** • <u>Breakfast:</u> Fortified Almond Milk Latte with Whole Grain Muffin • <u>Lunch:</u> Baked Sweet Potato with Cottage Cheese and Chives • <u>Dinner:</u> Miso Soup with Tofu and Seaweed • <u>Snack/Dessert:</u> Almond and Dark Chocolate Bark
WEDNESDAY	**Day 17:** • <u>Breakfast:</u> Smoothie with Kale, Almond Butter, and Fortified Orange Juice • <u>Lunch:</u> Sardine and Tomato Whole Grain Sandwich • <u>Dinner:</u> Lentil and Quinoa Stuffed Bell Peppers • <u>Snack/Dessert:</u> Baked Pears with Ricotta and Honey
THURSDAY	**Day 18:** • <u>Breakfast:</u> Quinoa Breakfast Bowl with Blueberries and Almonds • <u>Lunch:</u> Grilled Salmon Salad with Citrus Vinaigrette • <u>Dinner:</u> Roasted Chicken with Quinoa and Steamed Broccoli • <u>Snack/Dessert:</u> Blueberry and Almond Milk Smoothie Bowl
FRIDAY	**Day 19:** • <u>Breakfast:</u> Spinach and Cheese Omelette • <u>Lunch:</u> Mushroom and Tofu Stir-Fry • <u>Dinner:</u> Grilled Tofu with Stir-Fried Bok Choy and Sesame Seeds • <u>Snack/Dessert:</u> Cheese and Fruit Platter
SATURDAY	**Day 20:** • <u>Breakfast:</u> Baked Oatmeal with Apples and Walnuts • <u>Lunch:</u> Turkey and Avocado Wrap with Spinach • <u>Dinner:</u> Shrimp and Spinach Sauté with Almonds • <u>Snack/Dessert:</u> Orange and Yogurt Sorbet
SUNDAY	**Day 21:** • <u>Breakfast:</u> Ricotta and Honey on Whole Grain Toast • <u>Lunch:</u> Vitamin D-Fortified Soup with Chicken and Vegetables • <u>Dinner:</u> Grilled Tofu with Stir-Fried Vegetables • <u>Snack/Dessert:</u> Cottage Cheese and Pineapple Bowl

BONUS — WEEK FOUR MEAL PLAN

MONDAY	**Day 22:** • <u>Breakfast:</u> Scrambled Eggs with Spinach and Feta • <u>Lunch:</u> Tuna Salad with Lemon and Dill • <u>Dinner:</u> Turkey Meatballs with Spinach and Chickpeas • <u>Snack/Dessert:</u> Apricot and Almond Energy Bars
TUESDAY	**Day 23:** • <u>Breakfast:</u> Whole Grain Cereal with Fortified Milk • <u>Lunch:</u> Shrimp and Avocado Salad • <u>Dinner:</u> Baked Cod with Quinoa and Wilted Kale • <u>Snack/Dessert:</u> Almond and Blueberry Energy Bites
WEDNESDAY	**Day 24:** • <u>Breakfast:</u> Overnight Oats with Chia Seeds and Almonds • <u>Lunch:</u> Spinach and Mushroom Frittata • <u>Dinner:</u> Roasted Turkey with Garlic Mashed Sweet Potatoes • <u>Snack/Dessert:</u> Dark Chocolate-Covered Almonds
THURSDAY	**Day 25:** • <u>Breakfast:</u> Calcium-Fortified Pancakes with Maple Syrup • <u>Lunch:</u> Grilled Portobello Mushrooms with Quinoa • <u>Dinner:</u> Vegetarian Chili with Black Beans and Sweet Corn • <u>Snack/Dessert:</u> Frozen Yogurt with Mixed Berries
FRIDAY	**Day 26:** • <u>Breakfast:</u> Cottage Cheese with Pineapple and Walnuts • <u>Lunch:</u> Quinoa Salad with Kale and Grilled Chicken • <u>Dinner:</u> Beef and Vegetable Stir-Fry with Brown Rice • <u>Snack/Dessert:</u> Cheese and Whole Grain Crackers
SATURDAY	**Day 27:** • <u>Breakfast:</u> Tofu Scramble with Vegetables • <u>Lunch:</u> Sardine and Tomato Whole Grain Sandwich • <u>Dinner:</u> Grilled Shrimp Skewers with Veggie Couscous • <u>Snack/Dessert:</u> Baked Apples with Cinnamon and Walnuts
SUNDAY	**Day 28:** • <u>Breakfast:</u> Calcium-Fortified Waffles with Berry Compote • <u>Lunch:</u> Chickpea and Spinach Salad with Sunflower Seeds • <u>Dinner:</u> Herb-Crusted Pork Tenderloin with Roasted Root Vegetables • <u>Snack/Dessert:</u> Greek Yogurt Cheesecake with Honey Drizzle

WEEK 1: SHOPPING LIST

Proteins:
- 4 chicken breasts
- 4 salmon fillets
- 1 lb ground turkey
- 1 block of firm tofu
- 12 large eggs
- 1 package turkey bacon
- 1 lb shrimp
- 1 can of tuna (in water)

Dairy & Dairy Substitutes:
- 1 quart almond milk (fortified)
- 1 quart Greek yogurt (plain, low-fat)
- 1 container cottage cheese
- 1 block of feta cheese
- Ricotta cheese (small container)

Grains:
- Whole grain bread (1 loaf)
- Quinoa (2 cups)
- Rolled oats (1 bag)
- Brown rice (1 lb)
- Whole grain cereal (1 box)
- Whole grain pasta (1 box)

Vegetables:
- 1 bag spinach (fresh)
- 1 head of broccoli
- 1 bunch kale
- 1 bunch Swiss chard
- 1 large sweet potato
- 2 bell peppers (any color)
- 1 cucumber
- 1 head of romaine lettuce
- 1 bunch carrots
- 1 package mushrooms (baby Bella or white)
- 2 zucchinis
- 1 bunch fresh herbs (parsley, cilantro, or dill)

Fruits:
- 1 pint blueberries
- 4 bananas
- 1 pint strawberries
- 4 apples
- 2 oranges
- 1 pineapple
- 2 avocados
- 1 lemon

Nuts & Seeds:
- Almond butter (small jar)
- Chia seeds (small bag)
- Pumpkin seeds
- Walnuts (1 bag)
- Almonds (1 bag)
- Other:
- Olive oil
- Honey
- Balsamic vinegar
- Almond flour
- Garlic
- Canned chickpeas (2 cans)
- Tomato paste
- Whole grain crackers

WEEK 2: SHOPPING LIST

Proteins:
- 4 salmon fillets
- 1 package ground beef (lean)
- 4 chicken breasts
- 1 block of tofu
- 1 package turkey sausage
- 1 can sardines
- 1 dozen eggs

Dairy & Dairy Substitutes:
- Greek yogurt (1 quart)
- 1 container ricotta cheese
- Almond milk (fortified)
- Cottage cheese (small container)
- Shredded cheddar cheese

Grains:
- Quinoa (2 cups)
- Whole grain bread (1 loaf)
- Brown rice (1 lb)
- Whole grain tortillas (1 package)
- Whole grain pasta

Vegetables:
- Spinach (fresh)
- Broccoli
- Asparagus (1 bunch)
- Mushrooms (fresh or canned)
- Sweet potatoes (2)
- Bell peppers (2)
- Avocados (2)
- Kale (1 bunch)
- Cucumbers (2)
- Romaine lettuce
- Carrots (1 bunch)

Fruits:
- Strawberries (1 pint)
- Pineapple (1 whole)
- Oranges (4)
- Blueberries (1 pint)
- Apples (4)
- Bananas (4)
- Cherries (fresh or dried)
- Lemon (1)
- Avocados (2)

Nuts & Seeds:
- Almond butter (jar)
- Chia seeds
- Pumpkin seeds
- Walnuts (small bag)
- Other:
- Olive oil
- Balsamic vinegar
- Dijon mustard
- Almond flour
- Garlic
- Canned chickpeas
- Hummus (small tub)
- Honey

WEEK 3: SHOPPING LIST

Proteins:
- 4 chicken breasts
- 4 salmon fillets
- 1 block firm tofu
- 1 lb ground turkey
- 1 dozen eggs
- 1 can sardines
- 1 package shrimp
- 1 block feta cheese

Dairy & Dairy Substitutes:
- Greek yogurt (plain, 1 quart)
- Almond milk (fortified)
- Ricotta cheese
- Cottage cheese (small container)
- Mozzarella (block)

Grains:
- Whole grain bread (1 loaf)
- Quinoa (2 cups)
- Whole grain cereal
- Brown rice
- Whole grain pasta

Vegetables:
- Spinach (1 bag)
- Broccoli (1 head)
- Zucchini (2)
- Bell peppers (2)
- Kale (1 bunch)
- Sweet potato (2)
- Asparagus (1 bunch)
- Romaine lettuce
- Carrots (1 bunch)
- Mushrooms (1 package)
- Fresh herbs (parsley, dill, or cilantro)

Fruits:
- Blueberries (1 pint)
- Strawberries (1 pint)
- Bananas (4)
- Pineapple (1)
- Avocados (2)
- Oranges (4)
- Apples (4)

Nuts & Seeds:
- Almonds
- Walnuts
- Chia seeds
- Pumpkin seeds
- Other:
- Olive oil
- Honey
- Balsamic vinegar
- Almond flour
- Garlic
- Canned chickpeas
- Whole grain crackers

WEEK 4: SHOPPING LIST

Proteins:
- 4 salmon fillets
- 4 chicken breasts
- 1 block tofu
- 1 lb ground beef (lean)
- 1 lb shrimp
- 1 package turkey bacon
- 1 dozen eggs
- 1 can sardines

Dairy & Dairy Substitutes:
- Greek yogurt (plain)
- Cottage cheese
- Ricotta cheese
- Almond milk (fortified)
- Cheddar cheese

Grains:
- Quinoa (2 cups)
- Whole grain bread (1 loaf)
- Brown rice (1 lb)
- Whole grain pasta
- Whole grain crackers

Vegetables:
- Spinach (fresh, 1 bag)
- Broccoli (1 head)
- Sweet potatoes (2)
- Bell peppers (2)
- Mushrooms (1 package)
- Zucchini (2)
- Romaine lettuce
- Carrots (1 bunch)
- Kale (1 bunch)
- Cucumbers (2)
- Fresh herbs (parsley, cilantro)

Fruits:
- Blueberries (1 pint)
- Bananas (4)
- Strawberries (1 pint)
- Apples (4)
- Oranges (4)
- Pineapple (1)
- Avocados (2)

Nuts & Seeds:
- Almonds
- Walnuts
- Chia seeds
- Pumpkin seeds
- Other:
- Olive oil
- Honey
- Balsamic vinegar
- Almond flour
- Garlic
- Canned chickpeas
- Hummus

APPENDIX A

The Dirty Dozen and the Clean Fifteen

The Environmental Working Group (EWG), a nonprofit and environmental watchdog organization, reviews data from the U.S. Department of Agriculture (USDA) and the Food and Drug Administration (FDA) on pesticide residues in produce. Each year, they publish two important lists: the Dirty Dozen and the Clean Fifteen.

The Dirty Dozen list highlights fruits and vegetables with the highest levels of pesticide residues, making them the ones you should prioritize buying organic. On the other hand, the **Clean Fifteen list** features produce that has the lowest pesticide residues, making it safer to buy conventionally grown. However, even though these items are lower in pesticides, it's still important to wash them thoroughly.

These lists are updated annually, so be sure to check the latest version before you shop. You can find the most current lists and more information about pesticides in produce on the EWG website at www.EWG.org/FoodNews.

DIRTY DOZEN	CLEAN FIFTEEN
Strawberries spinach kale, collard & Mustard Green Grapes Peaches Pears Nectarines Apples Bell and hot peppers Cherries Blueberries Green beans	Sweet corn Avocados Pineapple Onions Papaya Sweet peas Asparagus Honeydew melon Kiwi Cabbage Watermelon Mushrooms Mango Sweet potatoes Carrots

APPENDIX B CONVERSION TABLES

VOLUME EQUIVALENTS (LIQUID):

US STANDARD	US STANDARD (OUNCES)	METRIC (APPROXIMATE)
2 tablespoons	1 fl. oz.	30 mL
¼ cup	2 fl. oz.	60 mL
½ cup	4 fl. oz.	120 mL
1 cup	8 fl. oz.	240 mL
1½ cups	12 fl. oz.	355 mL
2 cups or 1 pint	16 fl. oz.	475 mL
4 cups or 1 quart	32 fl. oz.	1 L
1 gallon	128 fl. oz.	4 L

WEIGHT EQUIVALENTS:

US STANDARD	METRIC (APPROXIMATE)
½ ounce	15 g
1 ounce	30 g
2 ounces	60 g
4 ounces	115 g
8 ounces	225 g
12 ounces	340 g
16 ounces or 1 pound	455 g

VOLUME EQUIVALENTS (DRY):

US STANDARD	METRIC (APPROXIMATE)
⅛ teaspoon	0.5 mL
¼ teaspoon	1 mL
½ teaspoon	2 mL
¾ teaspoon	4 mL
1 teaspoon	5 mL
1 tablespoon	15 mL
¼ cup	59 mL
⅓ cup	79 mL
½ cup	118 mL
⅔ cup	156 mL
¾ cup	177 mL
1 cup	235 mL
2 cups or 1 pint	475 mL
3 cups	700 mL
4 cups or 1 quart	1 L

OVEN TEMPERATURES:

FAHRENHEIT (F)	CELSIUS (C) (APPROXIMATE)
250°	120°
300°	150°
325°	165°
350°	180°
375°	190°
400°	200°
425°	220°
450°	230°

Made in the USA
Middletown, DE
26 March 2025